Introduction to Tobacco

Knowing more about Tobacco Abuse and Nicotine

I0420654

Health Learning Series

Dueep Jyot Singh

Mendon Cottage Books

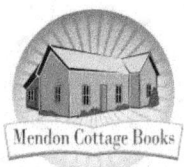

JD-Biz Publishing

All Rights Reserved.

No part of this publication may be reproduced in any form or by any means, including scanning, photocopying, or otherwise without prior written permission from JD-Biz Corp Copyright © 2015

All Images Licensed by Fotolia and 123RF.

Disclaimer

The information is this book is provided for informational purposes only. It is not intended to be used and medical advice or a substitute for proper medical treatment by a qualified health care provider. The information is believed to be accurate as presented based on research by the author.

The contents have not been evaluated by the U.S. Food and Drug Administration or any other Government or Health Organization and the contents in this book are not to be used to treat cure or prevent disease.

The author or publisher is not responsible for the use or safety of any diet, procedure or treatment mentioned in this book. The author or publisher is not responsible for errors or omissions that may exist.

Warning

The Book is for informational purposes only and before taking on any diet, treatment or medical procedure, it is recommended to consult with your primary health care provider.

Our books are available at

1. Amazon.com
2. Barnes and Noble
3. Itunes
4. Kobo
5. Smashwords
6. Google Play Books

Table of Contents

Introduction

The books in the healthy learning and gardening series published by Mendon Cottage books have given you a lot of knowledge about healthy plants, spices, herbs, flowers and trees, out there.

This book is introducing you to a plant which has been known as the good weed, tobacco, tabac and other local names, all over the world. It's usage is recreational and it is recognized in some form or the other, all over the globe.

The dried leaves of this particular plant is either pressed into powder, plugs, or it can be sliced into crumbly flakes. This book is going to tell you all about this plant, as well as its harmful side effects on the health of man and beast.

Tobacco is a native of North America, where the native Americans used it as a trade item. South Americans also knew it as an appetite suppressor. That is the reason why people of native South American tribes smoked these dried tobacco leaves when they knew that they would not have enough of food to fill their stomachs that day.

The tobacco which you are going to find all over the world is important and powerful nicotiana rustica, even though the chief commercially grown crop is N. Tabacum.

This preparation obtained from the drying of leaves is going to have it stimulant which is known as nicotine. This alkaloid is normally taken as chewing tobacco, snuffed as snuff or smoked in pipes, cigars, cigarettes, and also the Middle Eastern "shisha" which is flavored tobacco.

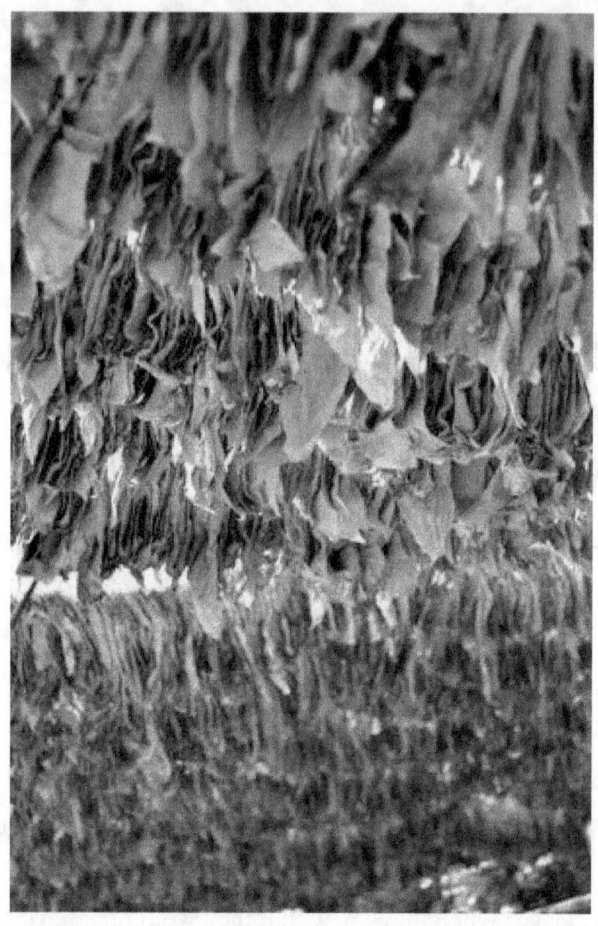

Believe it or not, tobacco is the world's greatest responsible factor for deaths which can be prevented. But as mankind has an innate and subconscious self-destructive instinct put into him by mother nature, tobacco products manufacture also happens to be a multibillion dollar industry, all over the world.

There are many countries like Cuba whose economies rest on the production of high-quality tobacco and exporting their products, all over the 16 corners of the earth.

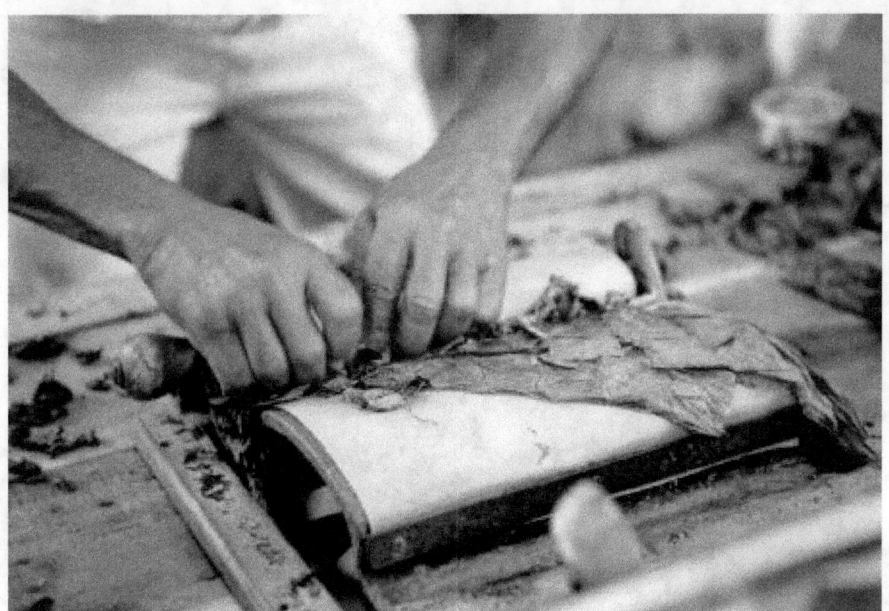

Tobacco was known to mankind for millenniums as seen in some archaeological digs in Mexico, Spain, Portugal, and other parts of the Caribbean, going back to 2000 BC.

The Native Americans used this stimulant in religious ceremonies, as well as in peace treaties. According to them, the smoke coming out from a tobacco pipe would go straight to God, along with the prayers, good wishes, thoughts and words spoken between two tribes with Him as a witness. During these ceremonies even children smoked the rolls of tobacco.

Tobacco was brought to Europe from the Caribbean by Spanish traders in the 16th century. Before that, I remember reading a story about the adventures of Sir Walter Raleigh of Elizabethan times who had received a quantity of tobacco from his adventuring friends, possibly, Sir Francis Drake and more roisterers Of the Seven Seas.

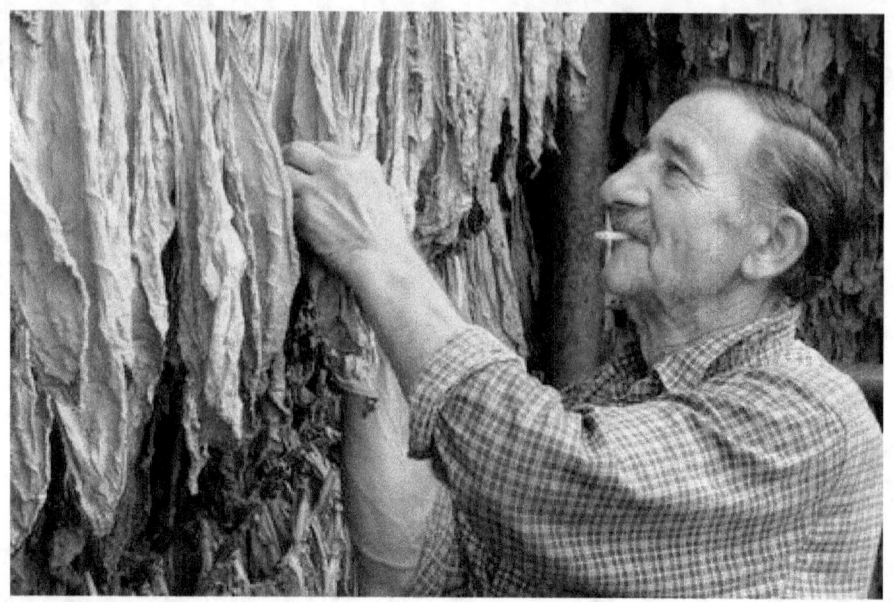

So one fine evening, he was sitting in front of his fire all relaxed and smoking his pipe. In came his servant, who saw that smoke curling up towards the roof and doused it immediately with a bucket of water poured all over his master's unsuspecting head.

This I think was the first example of a pipe being smoked in a European household. One wonders why we did not follow the practice of that wise servant and prevent this weed from choking out the lives of millions of people all over the world, even today in the 21st century. By 1700, all the European colonies had known all about the power of tobacco, and it was a major business industry.

The smoke was extremely harsh and was not inhaled. It was only later that milder strains of tobacco like White Burley and Virginia were developed, and tobacco smoking became popular in Europe too. Until then, tobacco was a popular and recognized trade item.

Naturally, it was only in the 20th century, when health related issues pertaining to tobacco were discovered and discussed by doctors and forums. But like I said, this is a multibillion dollar industry. Also, man has a habit of not listening to anything which is supposedly for his own good. That is why cigarette smoking and tobacco use in many forms still persists today, all over the earth.

I was looking at a beautiful miniature going back to the 14th century of a Mogul Emperor and a Rajput princess. Both of them were smoking water pipes! For them, it was an aristocratic pastime to be indulged in at leisure. But this is a well-known fact that in the Middle East, and in other Asian countries, the knowledge of tobacco was known to mankind for millenniums.

At that time, nobody knew it as a health hazard. In the 20th century, the USA was shaken with revelations about tobacco, causing respiratory problems and cancer. Instead of the government tamping down on tobacco use, it settled with the tobacco industry in an agreement with yearly payments! They could market their tobacco products supposedly in a restricted form, for a regular payment done to the government.

Nobody bothered much about tobacco as a health hazard at that particular moment. They were just glad that they got an opportunity to make up a Master Settlement Agreement, which said, all right, pay the government and the states so many billion dollars and keep marketing your hazardous products.

And *sauve qui peut.*

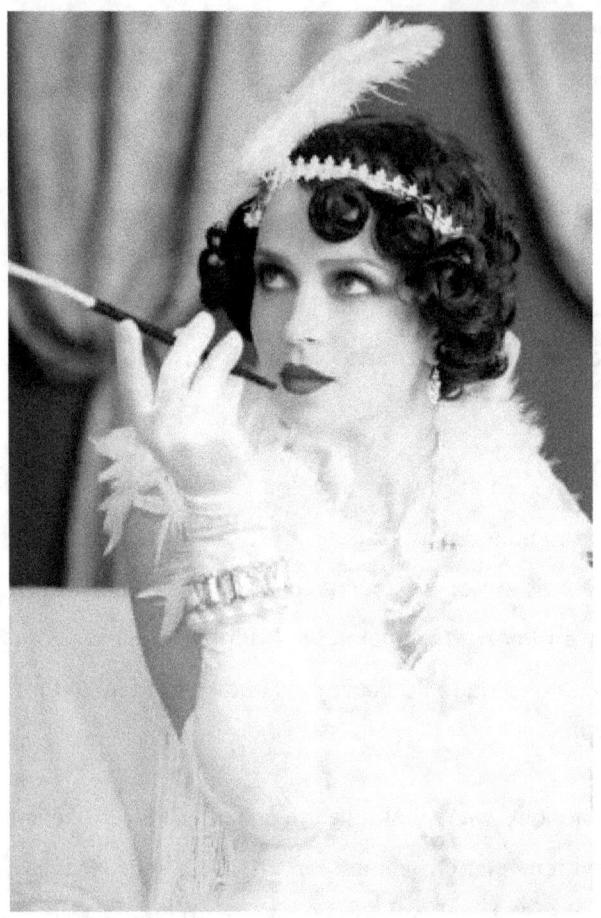

Tobacco companies began targeting women smokers In the 30s, after the First World War. According to them, smoking was stylish and milder cigarettes would not harm their health. All this was, of course, a false and misleading marketing and advertising stratagem.

My father remembers seeing a board in a train station – somewhere in the 60s and in the USA, – which said – *You Cannot Smoke Here. Not even Gold Flake* . These were the Wills Gold Flake cigarettes, which along with Camels were very popular in the USA since the 30s.

Naturally, the advertising campaigns for these cigarettes targeted adult males. And so we saw Malboro man still Malboro-ing in his own country. What the Surgeon General did not tell anybody that Malboro man may look the manliest of men, but if he continued smoking cigarettes, he would soon *be sterile.*

His woman when exposed to this continuous tobacco smoke, especially if he kept blowing smoke her way throughout the day would suffer from respiratory problems and bad skin. Especially when the nicotine content in the foggy atmosphere of a closed room got absorbed in the skin.

Their children, if any, would be born sick. That was because both the parents were not healthy. They would spend their lives trying hard to grasp for breath in a polluted atmosphere of thick tobacco smoke.

This was a fact well known to the ancients of the East. So that is the reason why tobacco usage, if any, was done very rarely and on special occasions. As time went by, the ancients began to understand the harmful effect of continuous tobacco usage, especially in smoked tobacco or inhaling the smoke.

That is why tobacco in any form is prohibited by a number of religions, including mine. So there is no question of my smoking ever or sniffing snuff or inhaling shisha.[1], even on a dare.

---

[1] My religion also prohibits imbibing alcohol- which is also a creed of Islam- but that is something which is not followed rigidly by a large number of my coreligionists. Going to bed without a nightcap or possibly drunk? Perish the thought! Yes, I have used the offensive term "coreligionists" because I definitely do not approve of drinking/smoking, especially when it is done to excess and has also

Even so, I have been suffering from a number of respiratory diseases since childhood. And why is that so? That is because even though nobody in the family smoked, everybody is in the neighborhood did!

Everyone did not mind lighting up and puffing away, because after all smoking was stylish, so manly, and it was a man's prerogative to have a cigarette hanging from the corner of his mouth, especially on social occasions.[2]

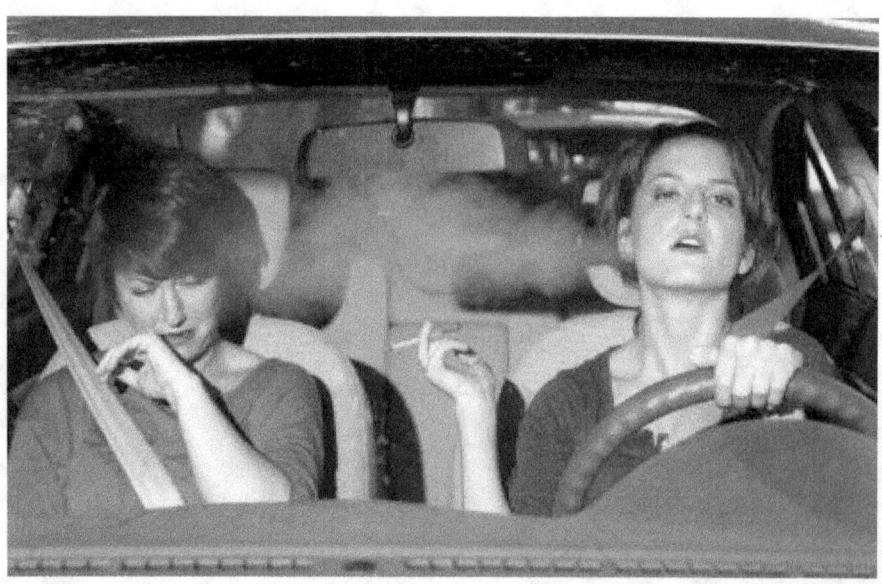

been forbidden by the wise ones. Not that I am fanatical about any religion and its principles and beliefs. Live and let live is my motto.

[2] . This was when the advertising campaigns for Gold Flake said – *A Touch of Gold – a Tribute to the Gracious People.* So who would not want to smoke such a stylish status symbol?

So we passive smokers got all the benefit of all that smoky atmospheres. And then came adult hood and jobs where nobody could possibly make a decision, go through a meeting, discuss anything, do anything constructive, or follow any official activity without cadging a fag and lighting up.

At that time, these colleagues were in their 20s, but they had started smoking in college. I am certain now that they are in their 40s, they are busy coughing their lungs out because at that time they were chain smokers.

Harmful long-term effects of nicotine? Forget about it. As long as you could concentrate and relax when you had a cigarette in your mouth, who cared? In fact, at this time, cigarettes were playing the exact role, Coke [cocaine] played for advertising professionals in the 60s. They were under the impression that Coke cleared up their thought processes, and it was not addictive. This was, of course, a falsehood. In my time, it was "oh, cigarettes, they help you to think. They relieve stress. You can relax with a cigarette in your mouth. Besides, it is not addictive. You can take it or leave it."

All of these statements also come under the Duh category and is the last ditch effort of a cigarette addict to justify his dependence on tobacco. Like Mark Twain said, "Quitting smoking is easy. I know because I've done it thousands of times."

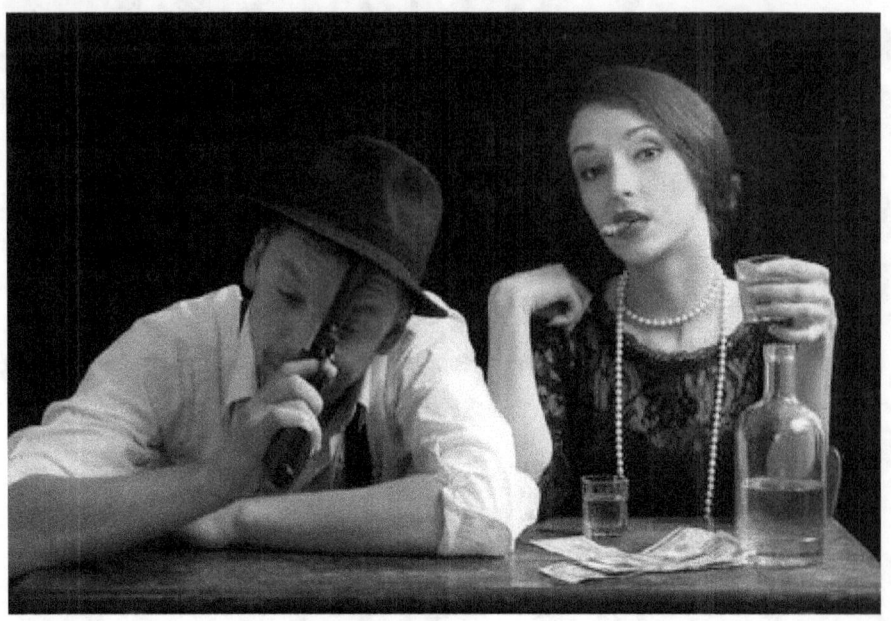

In the 19th century, especially in Europe, well brought up ladies did not smoke. This was supposed to be the domain of men and promiscuous women. So if I was in gay Paree in the 19th century, at Maxim's , and a pretty little lady bird caught my eye, I would just offer her a cigarette. If she accepted it, it also meant that she was willing to take our acquaintance, further.

Types of Tobacco

Down the ages, a number of tobaccos have come to be recognized as important trade items, economical wealth and cash crops. These tobacco types include and are not restricted to fire cured tobacco, which is aromatic.

You are normally going to get them in Virginia, Kentucky, and Tennessee, and are used in making blends for pipe tobacco, cigarettes, snuff, and chewing tobacco.

If you are in Syria or in Cyprus you are going to get the famous Latakia, the oriental version of *N. tabacum*. The leaves are cured, dried, and smoked over aromatic herbs, shrubs, and hardwood charcoal and fires.

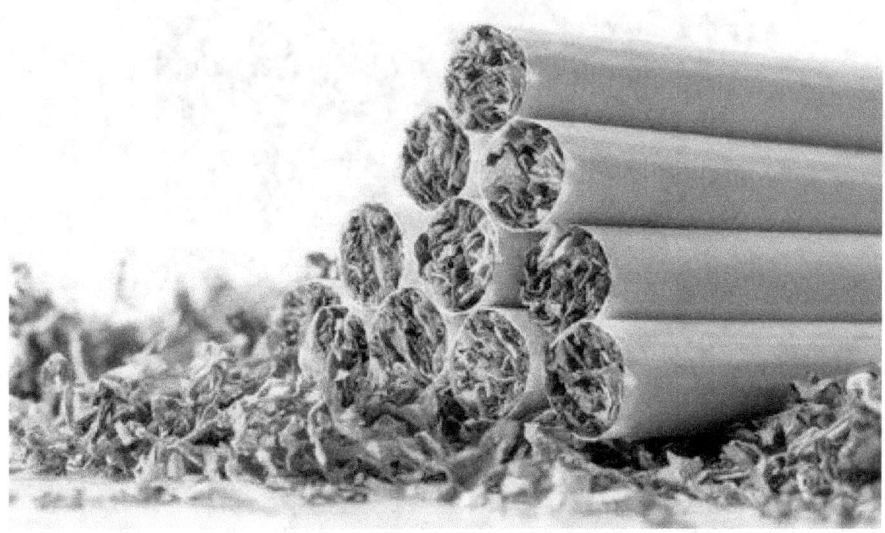

The popular tobacco grown in Virginia, was high-quality Bright Leaf. After the Civil War, this variety was still called Virginia tobacco, irrespective of the state in which it was grown. It is still a very important cash crop, especially when a majority of Canadian cigarettes are made up of hundred percent pure Virginian Bright Leaf tobacco.

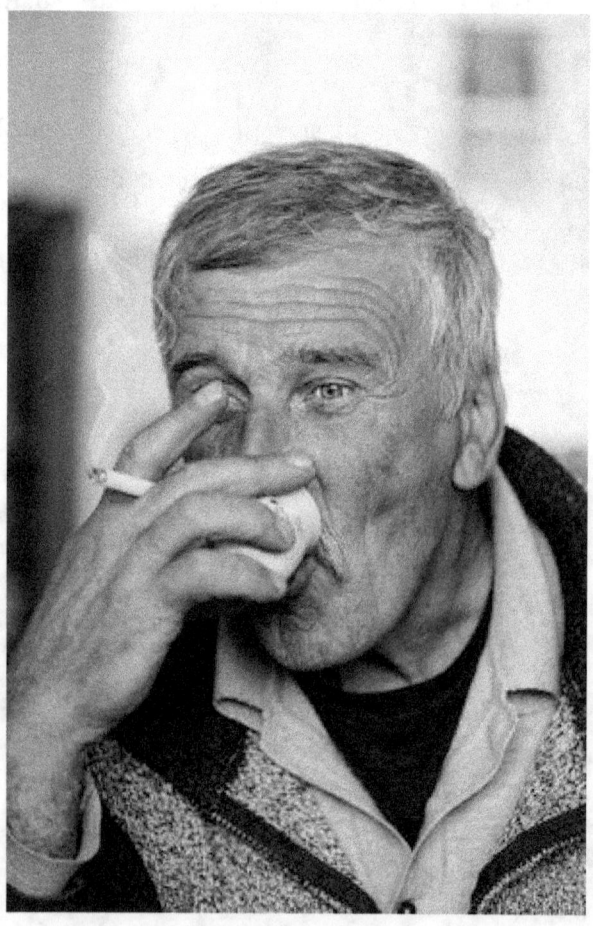

Cavendish is not a tobacco type. It is a procedure and method in which tobacco is cut and cured. The Cavendish mixture is going to be made up of Burley tobacco, Virginia and Kentucky tobacco to make up cigars and pipe tobacco.

In Iran, Dokha is the tobacco which is mixed up with herbs, bark, and leaves and smoked in a tobacco pipe, known as a midwakh.

Cuban tobacco is world famous, and it has been around since the day of Columbus as one of the most high quality trading crops in the world. The Romeo and Juliet cigar is a Cuban premier cigar, made iconic by Winston Churchill. The tobacco used in it is Criollo.

The Highly aromatic and small leafed variety of Turkish tobacco is grown extensively in Bulgaria, Macedonia, Greece, and Turkey. This is the tobacco which is marketed as oriental tobacco cured in the sun. The early cigarette brands were made from Turkish tobacco, but now it is restricted to pipe blends and cigarettes, with a mixture of Burley, and bright Virginia tobacco added.

Native Americans taught the early pioneers how to smoke tobacco, especially in pipes. Even though the Puritans called it The Evil Weed, they knew all about its commercial value and it was grown extensively in Massachusetts and Connecticut. Apart from this, native wild tobacco is found extensively in South America, the southwestern parts of the United States and in Mexico.

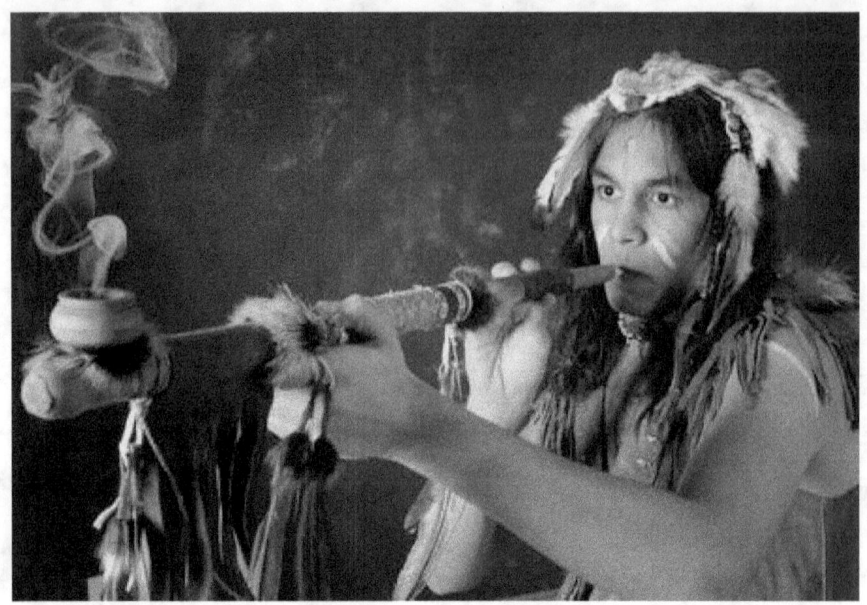

The pests were controlled with one of the strongest natural pesticides available to man – tobacco leaf water sprayed on the leaves and the plant.

If you are using a tobacco leaf solution as a pesticide, remember to cover up your nose well, because tobacco leaf inhaled in any form is definitely not conducive to good health.

When the plants are 8 inches in height, they are then placed in their permanent places in the fields. This cultivation is normally done during the rainy season, when a hole is made with a deer antler – admirable presumably basically a Native American tradition, using the easiest available implement practically and traditionally – and the seedling planted there.

So now you have two holes, thanks to the curved antler. Plant your seedling. Move 2 feet. Repeat procedure, continue until all the seedlings have been planted.

This method is still being followed in many parts of the world. Even today, harvesting is done by hand. Tobacco knives were used to harvest the stalks, and five – six stalks speared onto a sharp stick.

These sticks were then hung in the barn where the drying and curing was done. Around the 19th century, people began to harvest the tobacco leaves instead of cutting the complete stalk.

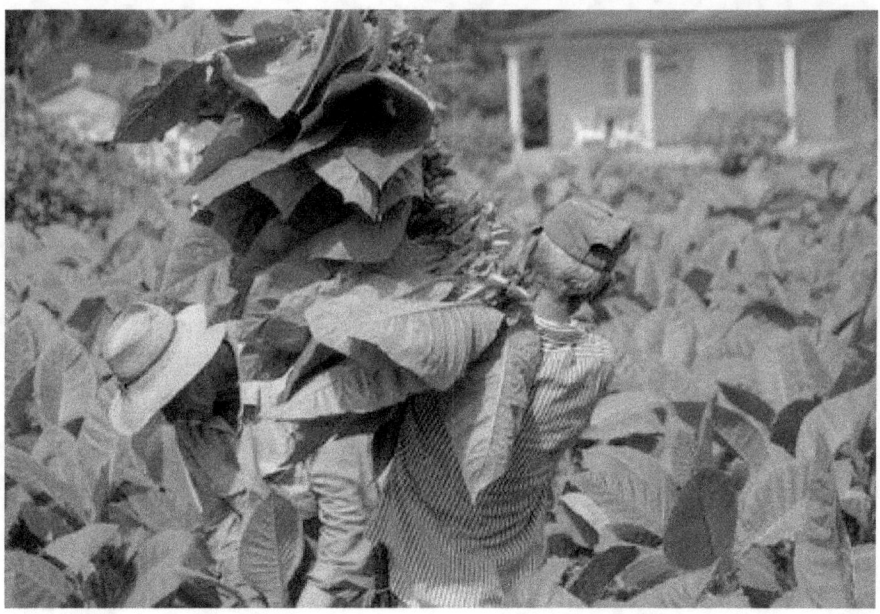

In this manner they could manage to get a number of harvesting from one plant itself, because the ripe leaves growing near the ground could be picked out individually. After that, the rest of the plant would grow in what could be considered to be a serial harvesting. Each harvest would be called the priming – the volado of the ripe leaves near to the ground, the seco priming of the leaves in the middle of the plant and the most powerful ligero priming of the leaves at the top of the plant.

To make sure one got this excellent harvest, the moment the pink tobacco flowers developed, they were topped off. That means the flower was removed before the tobacco leaf harvesting was done.

Even though tobacco plantations use harvesters to harvest tobacco today, in many parts of the world, harvesting, especially of immature leaves and topping of the flowers is still being done by hand.

Tobacco Curing

The slow curing process is going to add the flavor to the tobacco leaves. Incidentally, this is the time when the problematic oxidants appear in the leaves, which give rise to cancer and atherosclerosis. At the same time, the aromatic and fruity flavor of the smoke, which gives it that "smoothness" so well advertised by the branding companies is produced during the aging process.

Tobacco which has been cured in the air, especially in barns, and has dried for up to eight weeks is going to have a high nicotine content. It is going to have a mild and light flavor. The Burley and cigar tobaccos are processed in this manner.

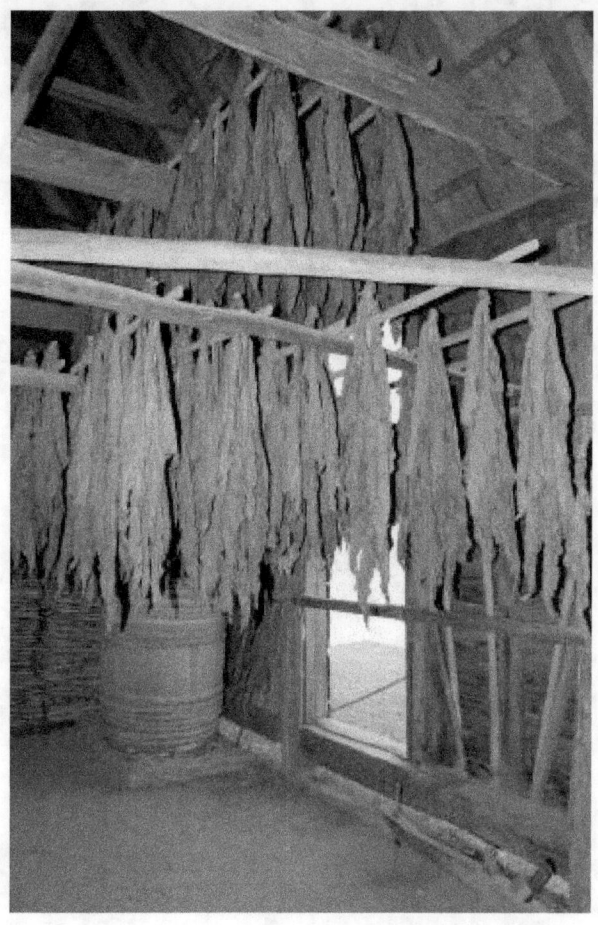

Tobaccos cured and smoked on fire can take anywhere between four days to 10 weeks for curing, depending on the variety of the tobacco and the procedure used. This is used to produce enough, chewing and pipe tobacco.

If you want tobacco, which is low on nicotine, try one which has been cured through a flue in a curing barn. Fire boxes are fed externally and the heat passes through the flue. This tobacco is not going to be exposed to any sort of smoke. One week of this procedure, and you are going to get a milder flavor, of which the smoke can be inhaled. But the nicotine level is going to be high or medium, depending on the amount of time used to cure the tobacco leaves.

Addictive Nature of Nicotine

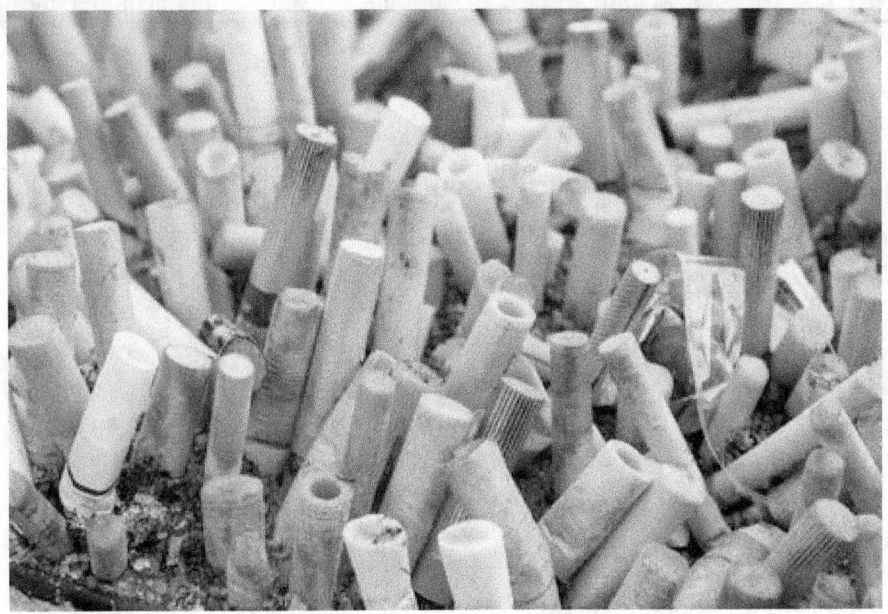

Nicotine is the compound responsible for the addictive nature of tobacco use. This insidious alkaloid is quite capable of changing the natural bio – physiological makeup of your body in such a manner, that the moment you do not get your daily dose of that particular alkaloid, you begin to feel uncomfortable.

Like other additives, this is also the reason why people suffering from nicotine deprivation suffer greatly from physical and mental withdrawal symptoms. That is because your body wants its daily dose of nicotine. I know about a friend who promised his kids never to smoke again, when he saw his very dear little daughter suffering from respiratory problems.

As he had been smoking regularly for the past 15 years, this withdrawal was very painful. First of all, his temperament. After that, his patience went out the door. Those three months craving for a cigarette were the worst he had ever experienced. Within a year, he had found himself feeling healthier and happier.

He was happy, his family was happy until his in-laws decided to pay him a long visit. Visiting him during this time I was shocked to see him with a fag in his mouth. He had started smoking again to keep his stress levels down. He also knew that if he had a cigarette in his mouth, he would not respond in an angry tone to some of his father-in-law and mother-in-law's more patent demands, opinions, and absurdities.

Well, you can consider this to be excuses to justify his going back to coffin nails, but even if a person has lots of willpower, it is rather difficult to stop smoking. That is because one does not want to go through the agony of bearing those withdrawal symptoms.

Tobacco Production Concerns

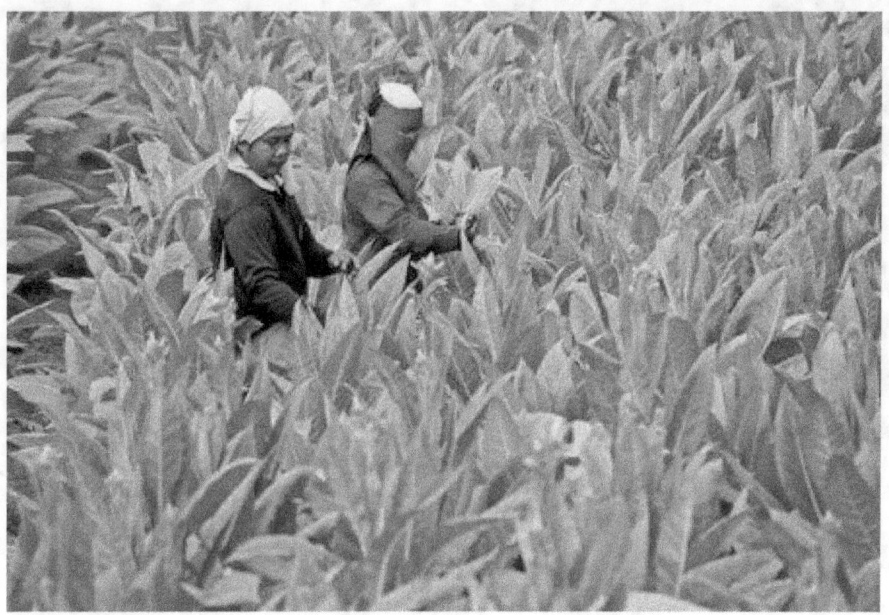

About 7,000,000 tons of tobacco leaves are produced globally. Many governments are making up to the fact that the labor used in the farms, especially those which are owned by families or in the factories, majorly consist of children.

These farms are more predominant in Malawi, Tunisia, Zimbabwe, India, Brazil, Argentina, and China, where child labor rules are not strict and they are considered to be the best labor for hazardous work.

Apart from child exploitation, these children are exposed to nicotine poisoning, especially when they handle the wet leaves. These poison is absorbed through the skin and is going to have about the same effect on one's brain and physiological makeup, as is obtained when one smokes about 50 cigarettes, over a given period of time.

Apart from that, the pesticides which are used to prevent pests from attacking the tobacco harvest are very strong and they can have a long-term harmful carcinogenic effect on these children

However, there are many countries all over the world, which couldn't care less about these health hazard. That is because apart from their economies relying on tobacco sales and export, major tobacco brand companies are encouraging the production of tobacco globally.

Japan tobacco, British American tobacco, and Philip Morris tobacco have leased facilities for manufacturing tobacco in 50 countries. They get their crude leaf supplies from 12 countries. Many Governments are also happy subsidizing such a profitable enterprise.

That is why there is a glut in the market today, and this extra surplus led to the dropping of the price of tobacco. So that is the reason why tobacco comes top in the **legal** products which you can smuggle with impunity, in the world today.

Tobacco curing also is leading to deforestation, especially in Brazil, where 60 million trees are cut every year to provide enough of Fuel for curing these leaves. Apart from that, extensive tobacco production in an area is going to leave the soil deficient in possession, nitrogen and phosphorus.

Forms of Tobacco Usage

So what are the different ways in which human beings get addicted to tobacco?

Chewing Tobacco Leaves

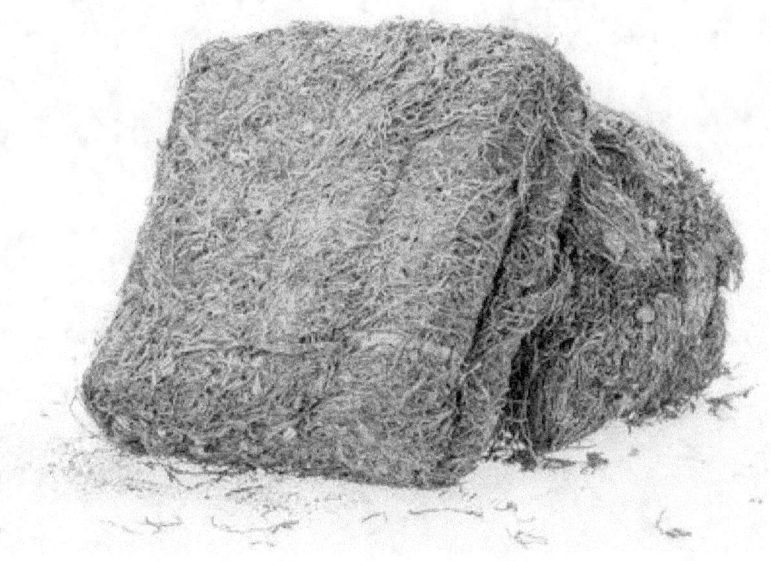

For millenniums, people have been chewing dried tobacco leaves where the leaves are shredded, chewed and made into a ball. This is then placed between the lower teeth and the bottom lip. This is going to stimulate the salivary glands, and that means that you are going to be spitting tobacco laden saliva, ever so often at the nearest available surface or any spittoon.

Just yesterday I saw the beginning of the movie *Zorro*, where the book and story is introduced by an old Western cowhand. After every five words, he went "squish", spitting on the ground. But this decidedly became not so funny after the first two minutes, when any obsessive statistician could have counted the number of times the spitting was done, 25 to 40 times, I believe in the four – five minute prelude to the story.

By then I had switched off to another movie, because this is definitely not amusing and two minutes of this activity goes a far way. So I did not manage to see *Zorro*.

Beedi

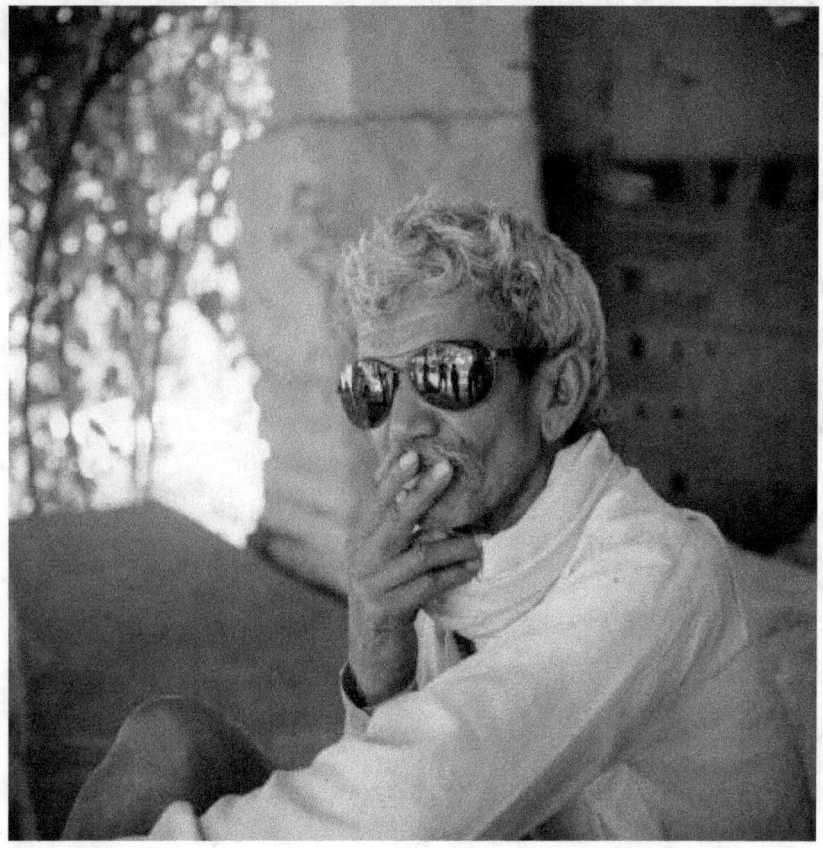

Beedi production is a multimillion rupees industry in India. I have seen rustic women smoking beedis wrapped up in a leaf, which is tied with a thread at one end to make a container in which to hold the tobacco. The leaf is called tendu, and every village is going to have a number of shops where you just go and ask for beedis to get your daily fix of nicotine at a cost of about two cents for 10 of these native cigarettes.

Tobacco Paste/Cream Snuff

Never heard of a tobacco paste, have you? Well, this is again an Indian invention of which I had never heard because it is a relatively modern 21st century, creation, targeting women consumers in Gujarat and Maharashtra. This is made up of a paste of glycerin, spearmint, tobacco leaves, camphor and menthol. The popular brands are Ganesh, Tona, and Ipco.

Apart from the tobacco fix, the consumers are really pleased that they have teeth free of dental problems, and shining, as well as minty fresh breath. *But they do not know that this is not a dental product, or a medicine for oral care. It is 100% tobacco-based product.*

You use it like a toothpaste upon your gums and teeth with either your finger or your toothbrush. It is not swallowed, and after five minutes, the mouth is rinsed with water. According to the manufacturers, this is an excellent way in which you do not need to internalize the tobacco, while getting the flavor of real tobacco without its accompanying side effects.

My view is – tobacco in any form, especially one which comes in contact with the gums is definitely going to have a future long-term bad effect.

Gutka

There is another typically Indian preparation – after all, this is the second largest producer of tobacco in the world – which is known as Gutka. It is a mixture of tobacco, herbs, flavorings, and betel nut, which combination is a nice and mild stimulant. That is the reason why college students and school students not knowing about the tobacco content began to buy it because of the high it gave them. One small packet for one dose costs about two cents.

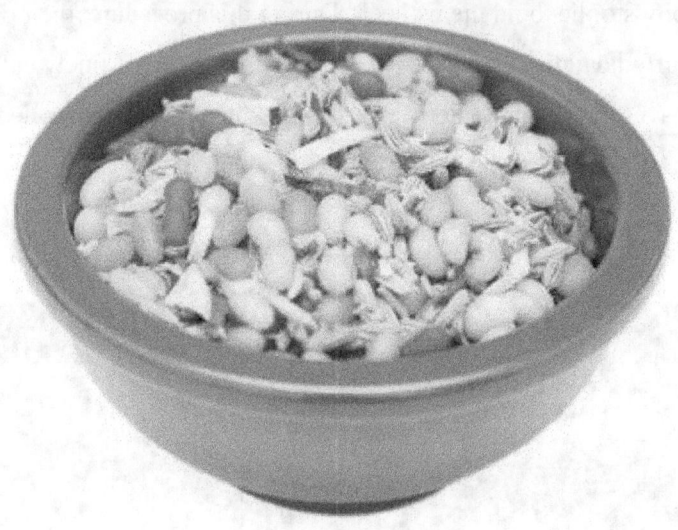

The government has now clamped down on the sale of this stimulant near schools and colleges and has channeled the production and sale to exporting this into countries nearby. Advertising and endorsing gutka is also being limited, even though the manufacturers do not advertise the fact that it consists of tobacco.

Cigars and Cigarettes

Havanas, Romeo and Juliet…, these bundles of tightly rolled fermented dendrite tobacco are iconic tobacco products. They are ignited and the smoke inhaled by the smoker.

After dinner cigars with port were part of high society traditions in the late 18th and the 19th century. In the 1930s, gangsters in Chicago, showed their degree of coolness by chewing on a cigar while ordering their men to give "that doity stoolie boid the woiks."[3] During this procedure, their dolls and molls puffed daintily on cigarettes which are made up of finely cut and cured leaves along with other flavors and additives, and then rolled into a cylinder of paper.

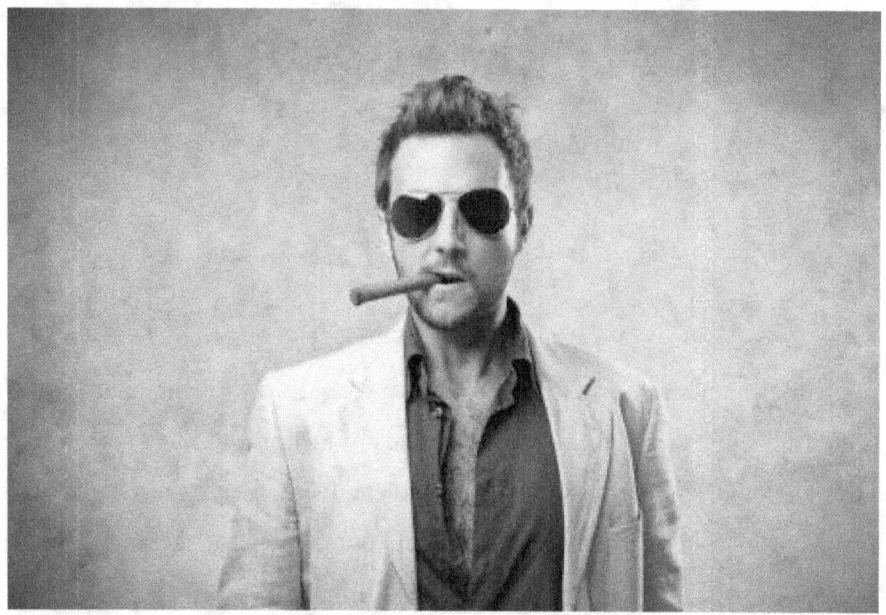

The cowboy of Western legend made his own cigarettes with tobacco paper and tobacco, he carried in his own pouch.

---

[3] Supposedly authentic Chicago Street slang of the 30s – read it in one of the pulp fiction, Penny Dreadfuls I like so very much.

The Water Pipe or Hookah

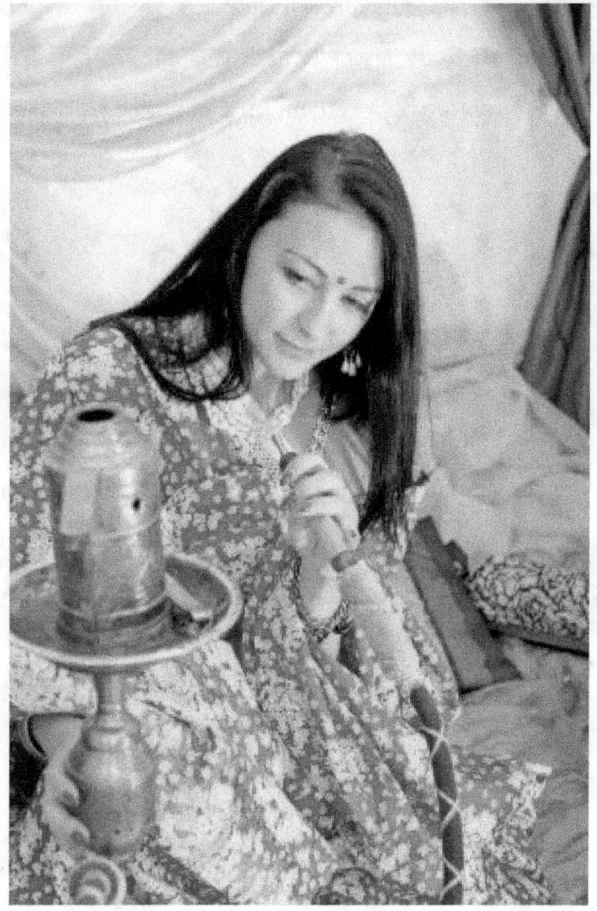

The water pipe is a glass based multi-stemmed or single pipe for smoking tobacco and has been in use in mid-Asia, the Middle East, Persia and India for centuries. The tobacco smoke which is flavored with honey, herbs, and other flavors, passes through the water and is filtered. It is supposed that this water filtration lessens its nicotine content.

Pipes

In the East, they have the hookahs. In the West, they have their pipes. The bowl was the chamber in which shreds of tobacco would be placed and lit. This bowl was attached to the shank, which was a thin stem. This stem or shank was covered with the bit or the mouthpiece. The smoke was then drawn through the pipe into the mouth and exhaled.

Kreteks

If you are in Indonesia, Java, and Sumatra and are a tobacco smoker, you may want to try this local cigarette. It is a mixture of cloves, tobacco and different flavors. The main aim was to get the medicinal clove product, eugenol, to clear up the lungs. But with the addition of tobacco, they are now just cigarettes producing nicotine to clog up the lungs! Now that is irony!

Snuff

This is a smokeless and ground tobacco leaf product which was snuffed through your nostrils. In Regency times, Masulipatam was a snuff obtained by East India Company traders to Britain from a city in the south of India. The Duke of Wellington used this snuff.

Social usage of snuff showed the acceptance of a person among his peers when he was offered snuff from the snuffbox of one of his acquaintances of equal social standing. And being offered snuff from the box of the Prince of Wales himself, well, You Had Arrived in Society with Bells on![4]

---

[4] Needless to say, Prinny never did that. In one of my favorite books written by Dornford Yates, one of the ancestors of the hero Berry [Bertram]Pleydell was presented a snuffbox by the capricious Prince as a token of his regard and esteem. That Regency gent immediately lost it to a highwayman Who Ordered Him to Stand and Deliver, that very night. And when the Prince asked for a pinch of snuff from the box he had presented to his friend Pleydell, on the instigation of another jealous member of the circle of course that could not be done. The Prince definitely did not believe the story of the highwayman.

Disgraced, Berry's great great grandfather left the Courts of idleness forever and retired to the country. And the box was found by his great great grandson, who had learned about this piece of family history recounted under the heading of *Put Not Your Faith in Princes*, as spoken bitterly by his cultured and well-educated ancestor.

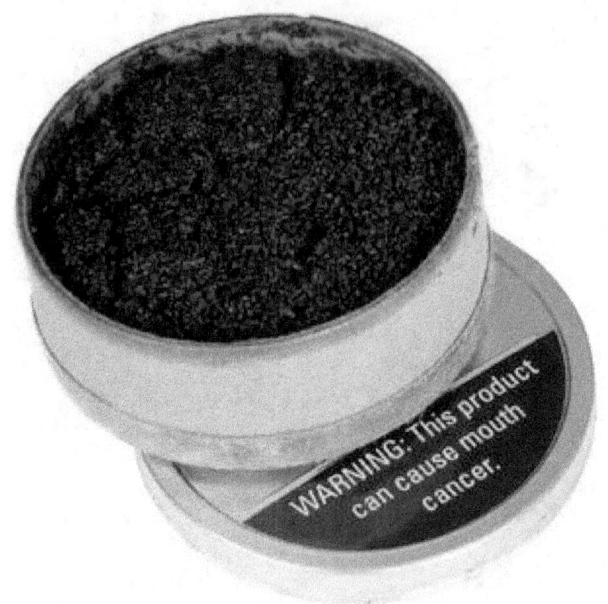

Tobacco to Heal

I have been talking about the harmful nature of tobacco, but like every natural product, it also happens to have plenty of healing qualities, when taken in moderation. I was astonished to know from my alternative medicine healer friend that tobacco has been used for centuries to cure diseases and successfully.

Since ancient times, in the East, dried and powdered tobacco and the leaves were used to clear up the lungs, nostrils and throat of accumulated phlegm with the help of inhaled smoke. The patient was made to inhale the smoke in limited quantities to clear up the system. Frankly, I would rather use saltwater in the Jal-neti method[5] of nasal irrigation to clear up my sinus, nostrils and throat. But then I do not touch tobacco. But the ancients did, and they also did not mind taking a hefty pinch of tobacco, in water to clear up their constipated digestive system.

Burns and Stings

A paste made up of fresh young tobacco leaves, crushed and applied to the burned skin would heal it. This is a traditional way of healing burns, but I would not suggest exposing your skin to ripe tobacco leaves – noticed I

---

[5] http://www.jalanetipot.com/

You may also want to read our book on this procedure by clicking on this link – http://www.amazon.com/Miracle-Water-Therapy-Oil-Pulling-ebook/dp/B00J1WTZ3G/ref=sr_1_1?ie=UTF8&qid=1441224058&sr=8-1&keywords=dueep+water+therapy

wrote young – for a long period of time. Prolonged exposure to tobacco leaves – let us say two years or three years handling tobacco leaves every day can cause tobacco leaf poisoning.

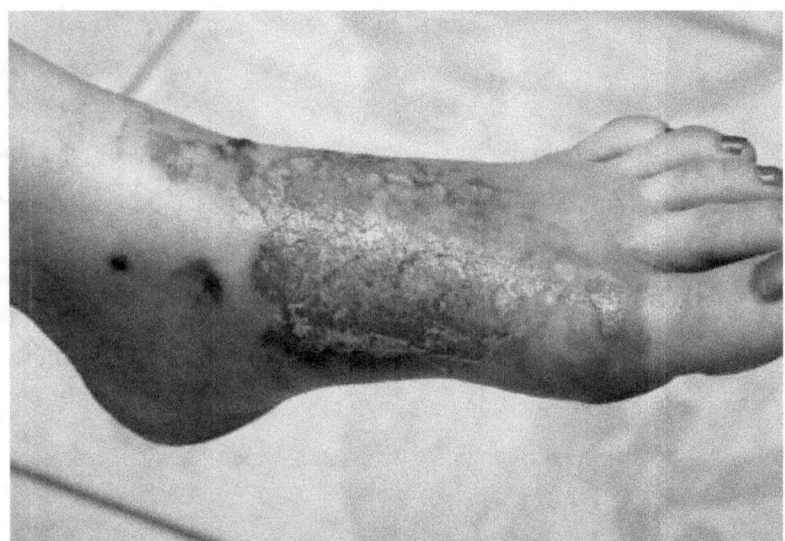

This is an occupational hazard for all the workers, working in Cuba, India, China, Brazil, and Caribbean countries where tobacco factories are common. Children may not be smoking this harmful "weed", but they are definitely exposed to the effects of those drying leaves, on their skin and due to inhalation. And as child labor is taken for granted in these areas, these children start suffering from nicotine poisoning when young.

Apart from being a burn cure, many over the counter remedies for stings are going to be tobacco pastes which are topical in nature. So if you are suffering from a bee, wasp, hornet, scorpion, or fire ants sting, just take out a cigarette and get rid of the tobacco in a cup. Add one teaspoonful of water so that you have a paste. Place this on the affected area for relief.

Joint Pains

This is a traditional remedy which has been in use for centuries to get rid of joint pains, especially in the knees. For this you need 120 g of powdered tobacco. It has to be soaked in 1 L of water overnight. Now squeeze the leaves, so that you get all the tobacco essence in the water and filter them.

Now you are going to take an equal quantity – 1 L of sesame or mustard oil. Add this to the water. Boil this mixture together until all the water has evaporated, and you just have oil. Now you have an oily infusion of tobacco leaves.

Place this oil in a glass bottle and store it in a cool dry place. Whenever you want to massage the affected area which is going to be two times a day, just remember to warm the oil, a little. It helps in better assimilation of the oil in the tissue, and reducing the pain. It is going to make your joints supple.

This oil is prepared in winter in the villages of the North in the Indian subcontinent. It is then sold as magic oil for your joints and knees. You may want to try it out on arthritis cases also. Believe it to work because it does.

So how long is it going to take for the pain to go away? Well, I said 1 L of oil. It is going to take about two months to finish the bottle, if you use it regularly twice a day. Massage for 15 minutes or more. You may find the warm oil, giving you instant relief.

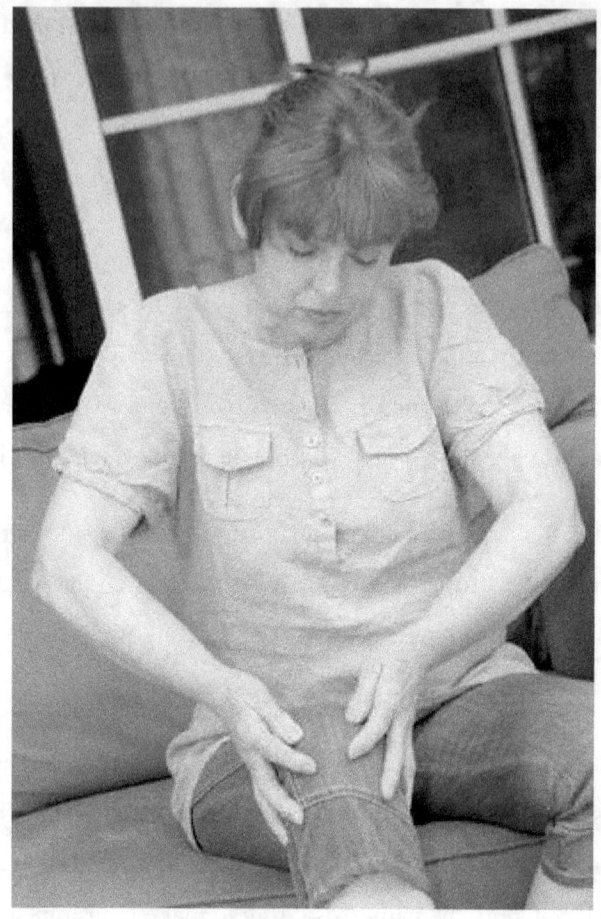

The pain will have gone away before the bottle is finished and you are going to wonder what to do with the rest of the oil! Place it in the sun, for two weeks and then you are going to have a long-term anti-joint pain, massage oil.

Tobacco for Tooth Problems

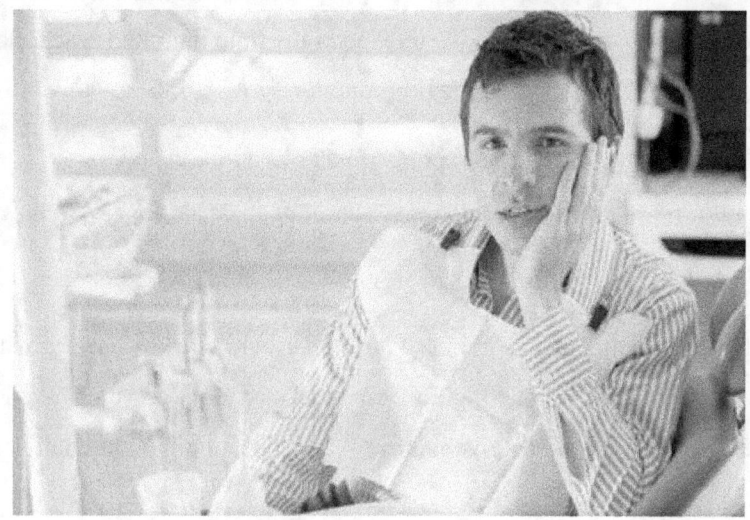

Whenever I see those stained teeth, obtained from chewing tobacco, I wonder how people considered tobacco for tooth problems down the ages. But unfortunately, that is true. Toothaches, cavities, bleeding gums, yellow scaling, and other gum problems can all be cured with tobacco powder.

Being a peripatetic sort of child, and traveling on all corners of the compass at the drop of a Posting Order, I have always enjoyed the adventure of traveling, especially on buses and trains. In many parts of the East, half of the fun in traveling is getting to different parts of the country where after every hundred miles, you are going to find a new culture, peoples and way of living. And that includes the items that they are going to hawk on the trains for all the travelers passing through their "land."

In some areas we looked forward to particular stations where we knew that we would get handmade velvet purses and pouches. In other places, we looked forward to buying handmade slippers and shoes. The vendors would jump on at that particular station, and spend the time it took to reach the next station in selling us their local products.

And at the next station they would take the train going back towards their destination. This sort of enterprise has been in existence ever since fast transport mediums came into being.

So naturally, we are always going to have a herbal remedies hawker who has his family members making up fresh stocks of tooth powders, ear ache oils, joint pain oil – recipe given above – and also an oil to cure baldness – alopecia – and dandruff.

As these secrets are well known to anybody who just asks for the recipe of any ancient herbal healer, here they are –

Take equal quantities of dried tobacco leaf powder and powdered peppercorns. Now, fry them together on low heat for two – three minutes. Mix them together with equal amounts of rock salt, and three powdered cloves.

This powder is used even today in many villages where they have not managed to get toothpaste in attractive packages. That is how they get rid of any sort of tooth problems.

Remedy for Night Blindness

Now this remedy has to be used with care, because you are going to apply .25 g of powdered tobacco leaves in your eyes. One paperclip weighing .25 g. I would suggest dipping the head of a pin in the tobacco powder three or four times and then shaking the powder off onto a piece of paper. Then apply this powder in your eyes and go off to sleep.

But before that, you need to fry tobacco leaves on a hot griddle and make them into a fine powder. Put them in a glass jar.

Night blindness is supposedly cured in less than a week, with this remedy. I am saying supposedly, because I am taking the word of an old and experienced shaman and I did not try it out, because I do not suffer from night blindness. But this is the night blindness powder sold on the buses and trains.

It is placed in a metal "soormchi" [6] – container – applied in the eyes with the applicator placed on it. Kajal, kohl, and other traditional Eastern beautifying cosmetics for the eyes are also placed in such a "surmadani". In olden times, these containers were made of silver and gold, and every beauty worth her salt had one. She normally applied it at night, so that by the morning, all the extra powder had been removed while asleep, and she woke up with kohl laden eyes, which would beguile everybody in the vicinity for the whole day.

---

[6] . This is how it normally looks. https://www.etsy.com/in-en/market/surmadani

You do not need to buy it unless you are totally addicted to kohl!

The one which I inherited from grandma, is made up of some metal, of which I do not know the name, but it is more than 120 years old.

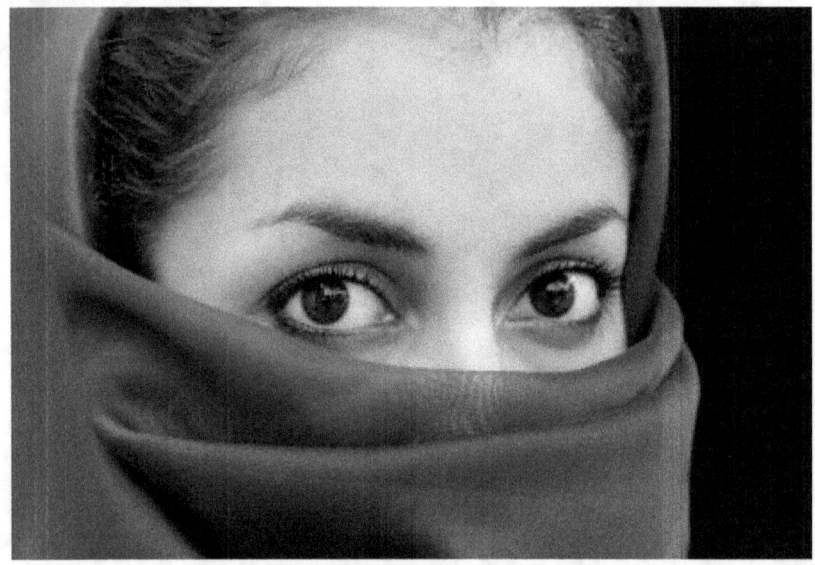

These beautiful kohl laden eyes are never going to suffer from night blindness, if the old and proven remedy of tobacco powder is used at night.

Earache and Ear Problems –

Living in moisture filled mountaineous areas for a major portion of my life, I used to suffer a lot from Otitis externa, which meant an infected ear as a kid. That meant I had to go every third day to the hospital and get my ears cleaned out of the infection, and the accumulated wax. After that, the doctor used to put in some ear drops, but he never ever told me to stop swimming!

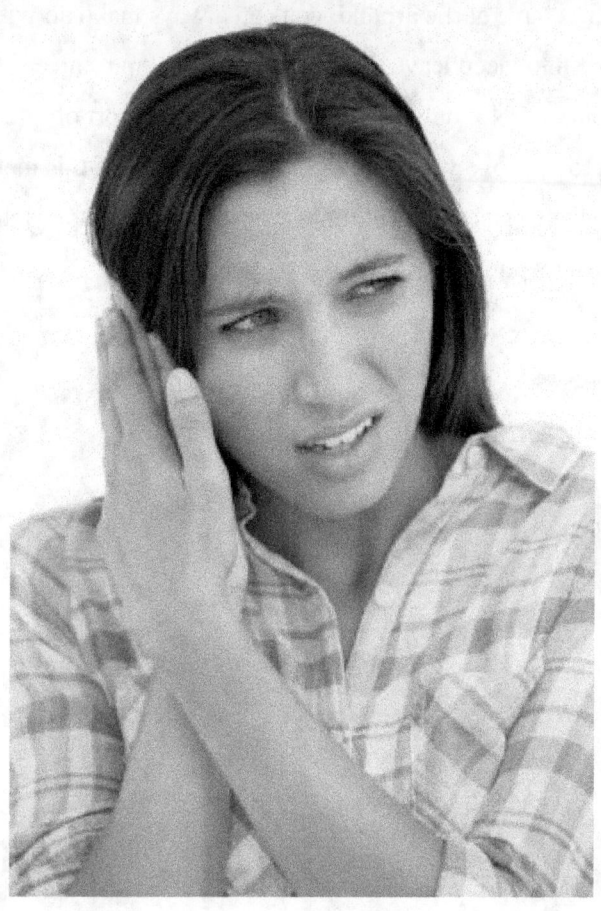

Water in ears, and not dried out properly, and voila, ear infection raging within two days again. Until my grandmother got really annoyed at my yowling in pain every night – looking for an ear bud to get rid of the infected accumulation – and tried her own herbal remedy of one teaspoonful of mustard oil in which she had burnt two cloves of garlic.

Two drops in each ear with warm oil, three times a day, and the infection cleared up within three days, to come back only very rarely as an adult when I forgot to dry the inside of my ears after swimming.

So if you do not have garlic around, you can always make do with juice from some fresh tobacco leaves. Just grind them and put three – four drops straight in your ear. Not only is going to clear up any sort of infection, but it is also going to improve your hearing. Try it out because this method has been used in places since ancient times where tobacco usage is the norm instead of the exception.

Alopecia – baldness

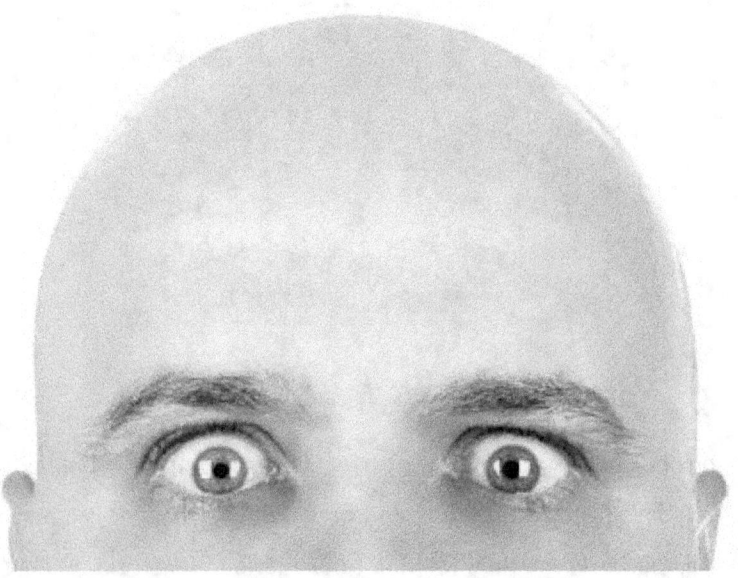

Here is a time proven remedy which can get your hair back, though it is going to take anywhere between six months to one year. That is the time it is going to take for the hair follicles to decide they are getting enough of nourishment to replenish themselves, and they need to start growing again.

For this you are going to need a bottle of coconut oil, or any oil with which you moisturize your hair. You can also use olive oil, sesame oil, mustard oil, and any other oil as long as it is not refined and it has its original strength.

Now get some good quality tobacco – 25 g –and powder the leaves thoroughly. Keep adding coconut oil to this mixture until the leaves are thoroughly drenched.

Close the lid, of this air tight container and allow the tobacco to seep in the oil for three days. Normally, this is done in a glass vessel, or in a metal vessel. I do not admire plastics, much, especially when I am seeping anything.

After three days, squeeze the powder so that any remaining extract is extracted in the oil. Filter the oil, put it in the glass bottle, and use it at night before going to sleep, on the bald spot, massaging slowly.

This remedy isn't for drinking!

Tips for Controlling That Craving

Everybody knows that you need a lot of willpower to get rid of that craving for a coffin nail. Unfortunately, a large percentage of people out there do not have that sort of Will Power. That is because the moment they sit down and start to do some work which needs a bit of concentration, they automatically reach out for a fag.

Here is some tips and techniques, which can help you get rid of that addiction. The first one, which I have seen working is chewing fennel seeds.

Fennel

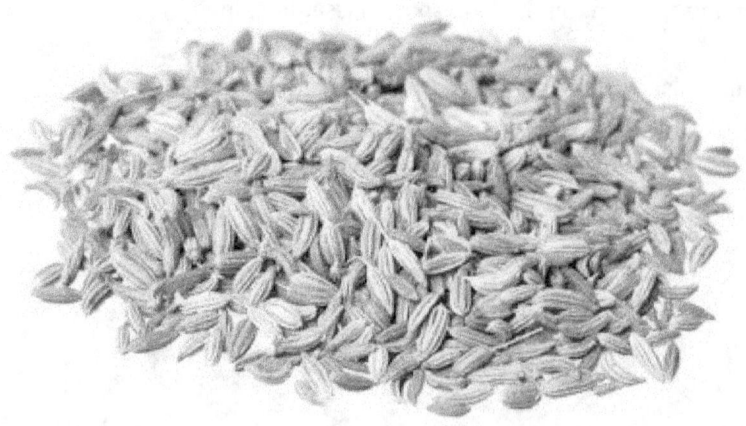

I saw this herb being used in detoxification and de-addiction centers, where they were using a mixture of ancient remedies as well as traditional remedies to get rid of nicotine as well as alcohol dependence.

You are now going to be changing your lifestyle.

Diet Change

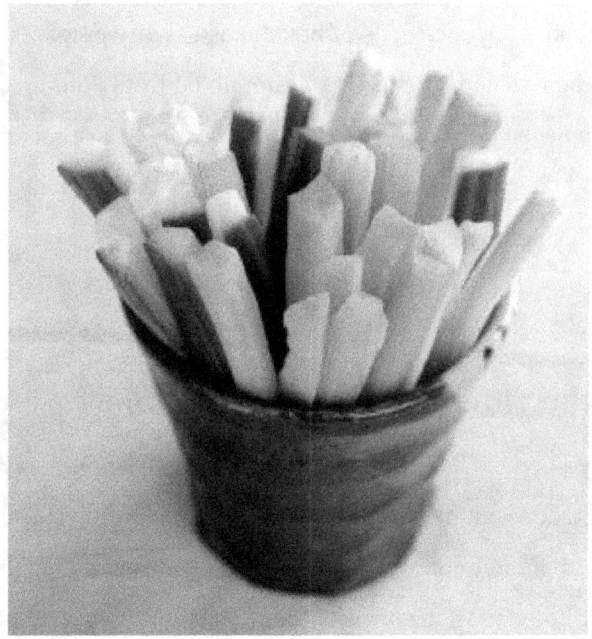

So firstly, make sure that you remove fatty foods, chocolates, coffee, sugar, and alcohol from your diet for the first two weeks. These foods stimulate your craving for nicotine because they happen to be a bit addictive themselves.

Before starting work or anything which is going to need a little bit of concentration, cut up a number of carrot, cucumber sticks, and celery sticks. The moment you want to reach for a cigarette, put them in your mouth.

Not only are you going to stimulate the taste buds which wanted nicotine with another food , but these are definitely a healthier substitute. Alternate the bites with sips of water or fresh lemon juice with a spoonful of honey.

Your diet is going to be vegetarian for the duration, while you are getting rid of the withdrawal symptoms.

Also, your intake of acidic foods of bread, pasta, dairy products, tea, and coffee has to be reduced drastically or eliminated from your diet. These are going to be replaced with sprouts, nuts, fruit, Lima beans, raisins, vegetables and beets, which are excellent to reduce that craving and getting you to give up smoking.

Boost up the Vitamin C and Honey Intake

Let me give you one insider tip. If you are a chronic smoker, increase your vitamins C intake. That means start eating more grapefruits, oranges and lemons. This is going to boost up your immunity system. It is also going to detoxify your body of all the toxins accumulated due to the nicotine buildup.

If you are not a diabetic and you can take honey, start adding it to all your sweet food items, in order to reduce the craving. Fresh juice with a spoonful of honey is going to rejuvenate your body.

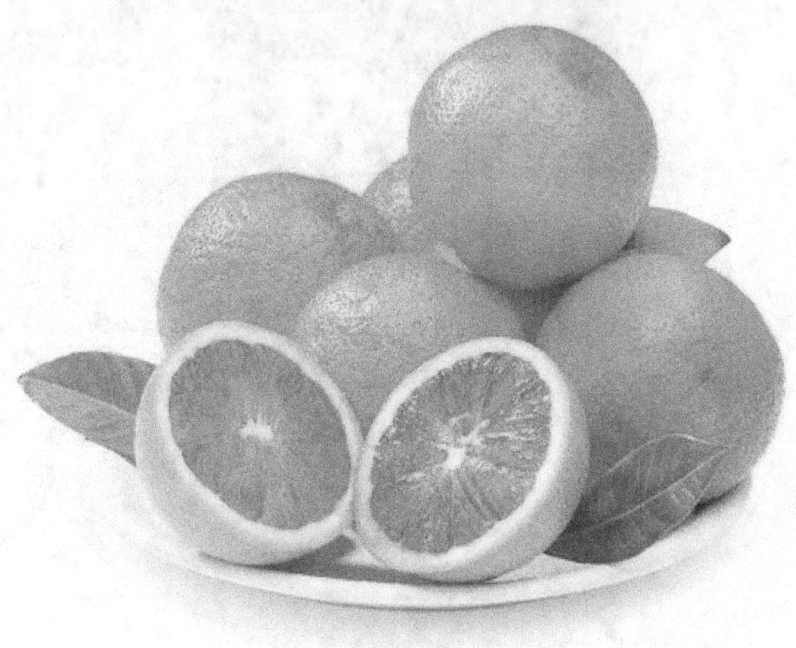

Other Things on Which to Chew

One of my friends gave me this tip. The moment she wanted a cigarette, she would just take out a salty piece of snack and crunch it. If she did not have anything salty in snack form ready at hand, she had a little bit of cooking/rock/black salt in a packet. Just a touch of it on the tongue's tip and the craving went away instantly. Try it out.

Try chewing licorice. It is sweet, and helps as a substitute for a cigarette, especially when you are just craving for a smoke. Also licorice is good as a soother for that hacking cough brought on by smoking.

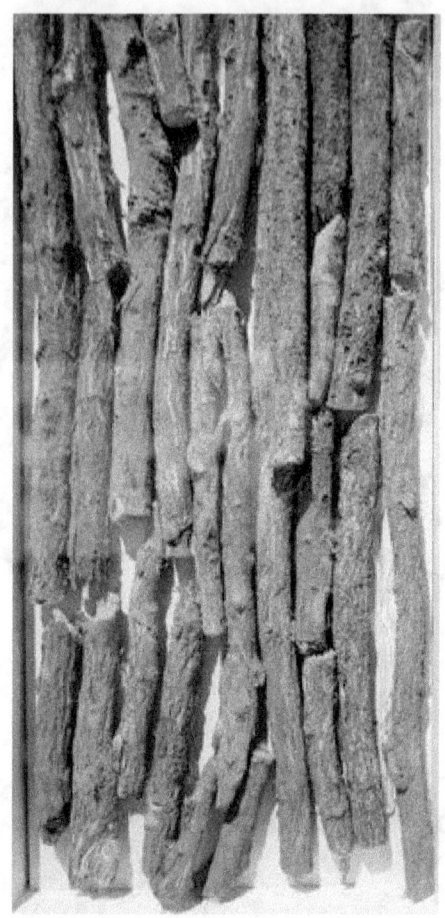

Licorice Root

In Eastern villages where people are addicted to chewing tobacco, they are instead asked to chew upon stubs of sugarcane.

I Will Stop at One...

Remember that you are substituting one flavor and taste for another. But what happens when you are in the middle of a meeting, and you just want, you just cannot do without a cigarette, and there is nothing at hand.

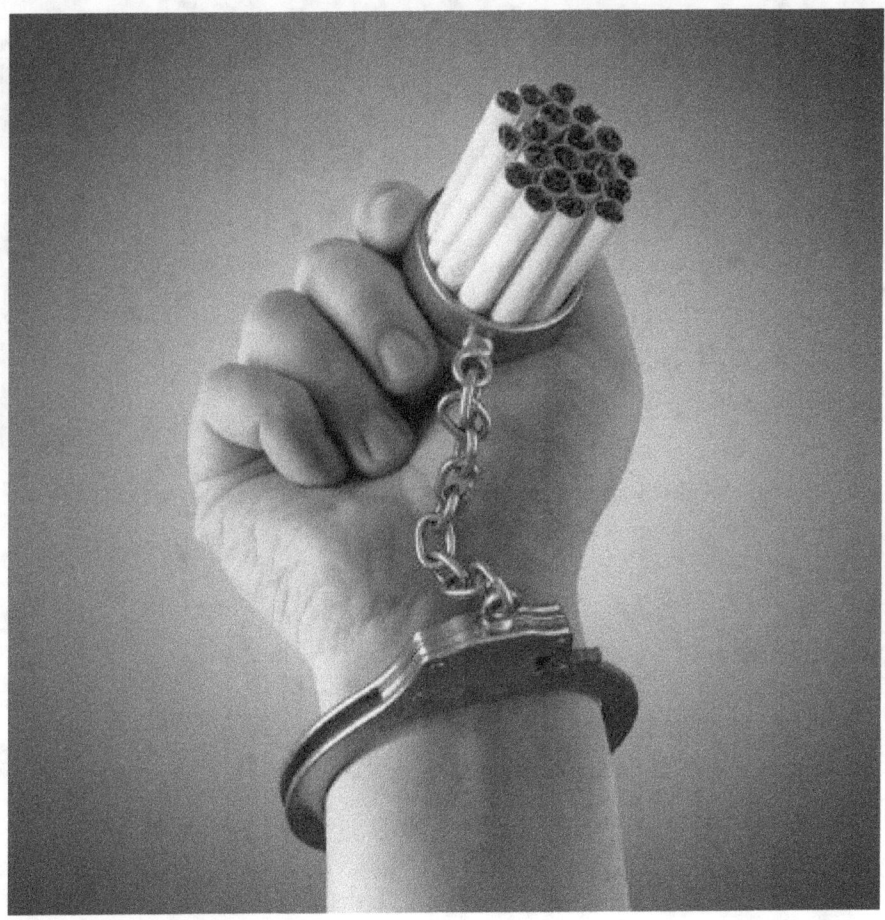

You promise yourself that you just need one and you are going to stop at one. Cannot be done. That one is going to lead to just one more and there you are, you are polluting the atmosphere with cigarette smoke with the people all around you, too polite to tell you to stop stinking up the premises.

This is when you need a little bit of willpower. Just tell yourself that you can manage to wait 10 minutes before you give in. Start doing something creative, immediately which is going to occupy your hands and mind so that you do not have the time to reach for a cigarette.

This was a tip told to me by a chronic smoker. He said that the moment he had to think of something when his hands were not doing something actively, his mind said – so where is the cigarette. But the moment he started concentrating on something really problematic and potentially tiresome, he found that craving being derailed. His subconscious mind kept prodding, cigarettes, cigarettes, but concentration was fixed on the duty he needed to do right now. And he quit smoking after being a chronic smoker for 20 years.

Now, I consider this to be a real show of the power of mind over matter.

Identifying Triggers

There are number of triggers which are going to bring about that urge for smoking. Do you begin smoking when you watch TV? Are you a smoker when you are driving the car, or waiting for someone? When you have identified these main triggers, try to avoid them as far as possible.

That is because your mind associates cigarettes with these particular activities during the years gone by. Your mind has to be channeled into some other thought related to that particular activity. Try chewing mint gum when watching TV. Or just snack off carrot slices.

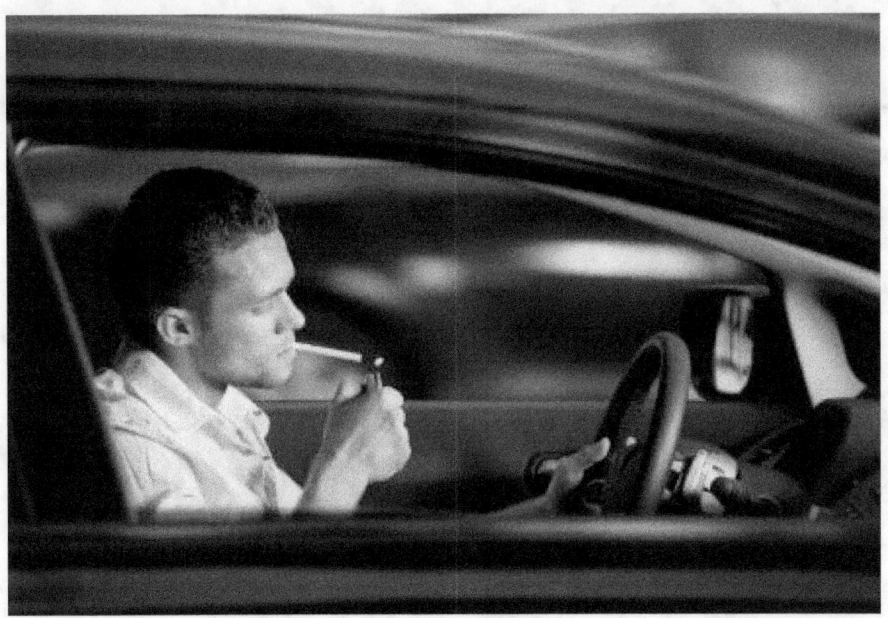

If you light up when you are waiting for a phone call, I would suggest placing a ball pen on your table. The moment you want to smoke, just put that ball pen in your mouth and bite hard on it. It is going to keep your mouth occupied. Also keep your hand occupied by doodling on a piece of paper, especially cartoons of animals smoking cigarettes and then coughing away.

Exercise and Occupying Your Mind and Hands

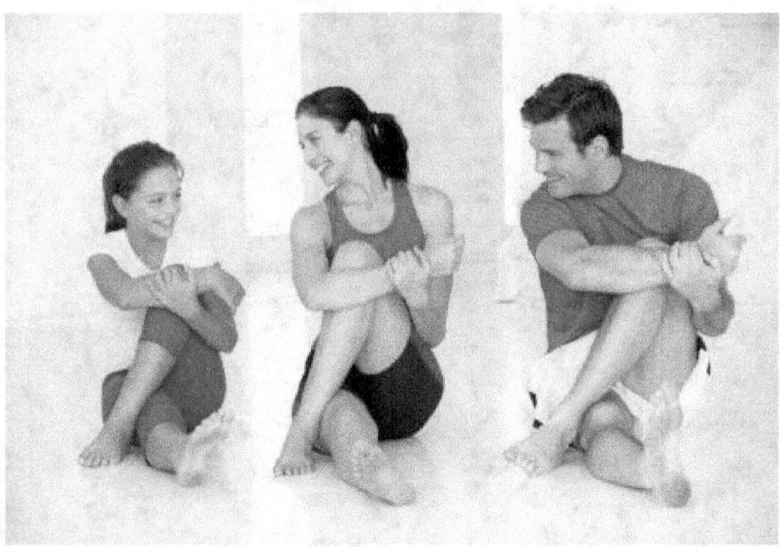

A sedentary lifestyle is one of the reasons why so many people smoke cigarettes. If you are out in the air, doing something physical and active, especially using both hands, you may find the tobacco craving going away. It has been sent to fully proven that 30 minutes of any sort of physical exercise or activity gets rid of that craving.

Why is that so? That is because the body has begun pumping in healthy secretions like adrenaline, etc. to keep the oxygen supply moving when your lungs are starved for air, especially if you are climbing up the stairs, running on a piece of carpet, or even jogging.

If you do not like any sort of physical activity which would need a little bit of exertion, – join the gang, including I, you can never get me to exercise involuntarily or voluntarily; been through that sort of rigorous, disciplined and strict torture during athletics training at college and promised myself never again – try something else. Start scrubbing up the house or filing away paperwork. You can also try needlework or anything else, which occupies your hands. Keep your mouth occupied with chewing gum or with talking or singing!

Stress Busting

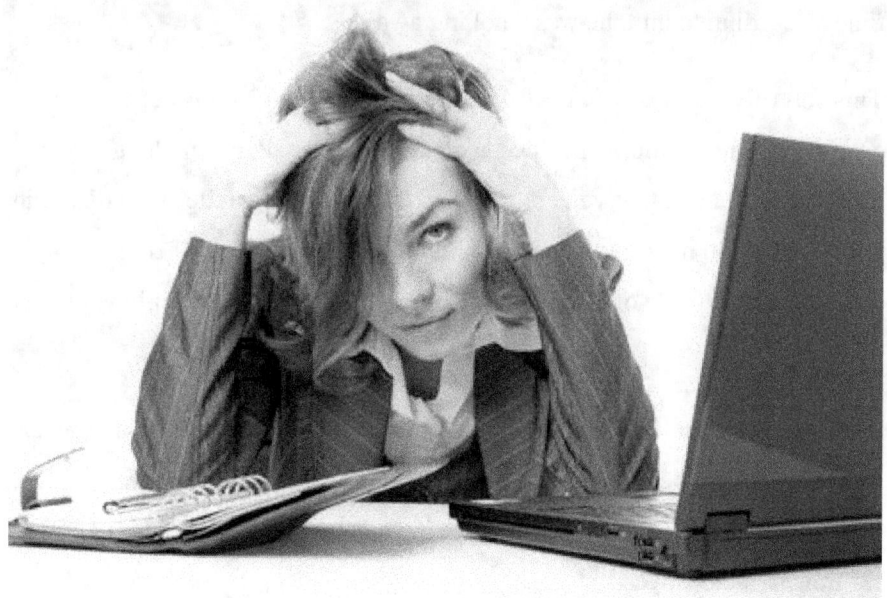

These are different ways in which you are going to distract yourself. You started smoking in order to get rid of that stress and tension. Now you have reached this stage when stopping smoking is causing you stress!

Meditation, deep breathing exercises, relaxation and yoga is excellent to get rid of all that stress and relaxing your mind.

I remember a Maurice Walsh book in which the hero is so busy planning a strategy that he puts an unlit pipe in his mouth, and goes out for a walk. Half-an-hour later he wakes up from his trance and asks his friends accompanying him how he got there.

His friend explains this phenomenon to the heroine by telling her that in his mind he is puffing away at his pipe. He is smoking it and thinking at the same time. And he has worked out the solution to the problem. During this time, according to him, he was smoking away!

This sort of visualization can also be done by a person who is deep in concentration on a job, which needs mental exercise. Put something in your mouth and imagine that you are smoking a pipe or a cigarette. Visualize it in your mind. You may find yourself thinking that this is true, when in reality you just have a piece of carrot or an empty pipe or even a pencil in your mouth!

Remember a person trying to get rid of any sort of addiction is going to need lots of support. There are plenty of online forums, especially where you can read amusing stories about how people have managed to tackle their craving for this pernicious weed.

BBC's Sherlock uses a nicotine patch, when the original Sherlock stuck a pipe in his mouth or sniffed cocaine. You can try these over the counter replacement therapies.

Remember to appreciate each day, which has passed by without you smoking. That means you have taken a major step in beating this craving for tobacco.

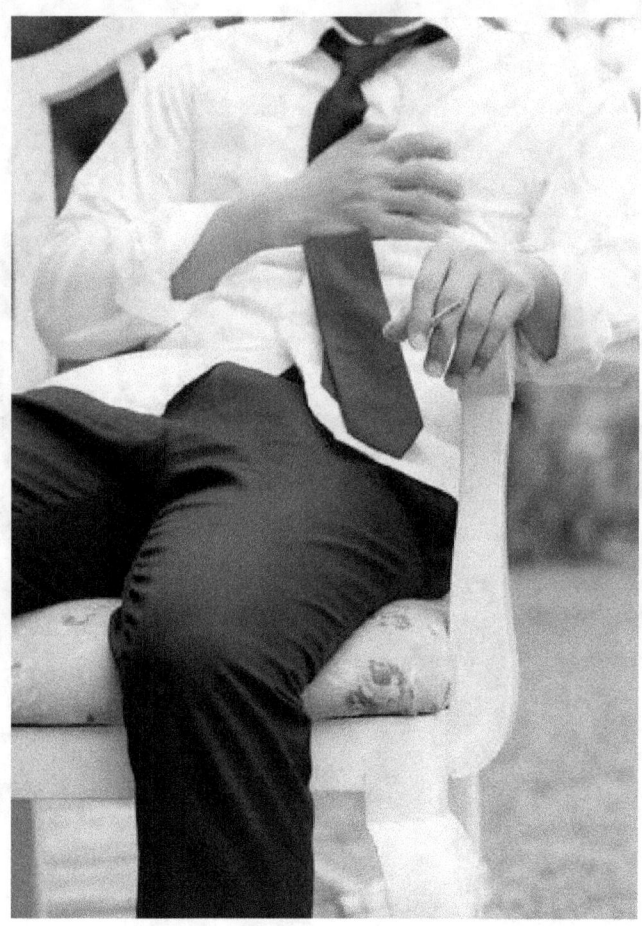

Conclusion

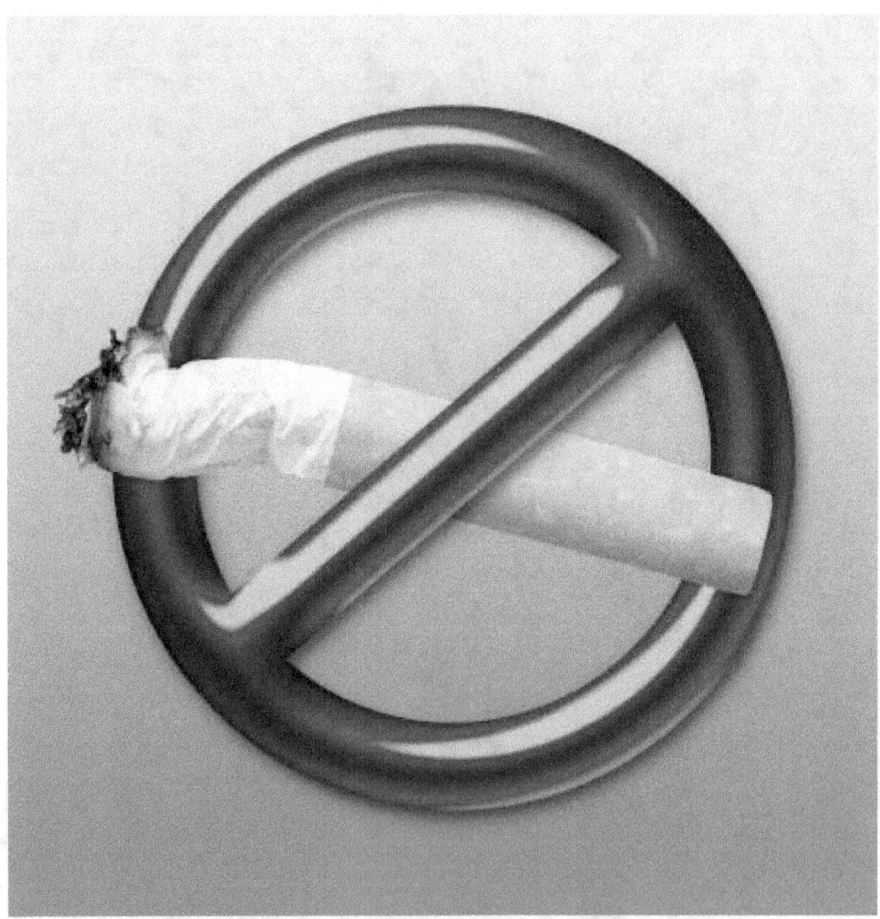

The only country in the world today where sales of tobacco is illegal is Bhutan. The rest of the world has antismoking and boycott tobacco campaigns and forums, but they are definitely not going to have any effect, as long as multibillion-dollar tobacco producing companies keep getting trade subsidies from governments.

Apart from that, vigorous advertising has brought about the Association of cigarette smoking and cigar smoking to be a particularly manly and virile activity done by men with style, distinction, status, social standing and grace. Many of these campaigns, like alcohol ads and car ads, want to show women being attracted by men who smoke one particular brand of cigarette.

Not only is this demeaning to women as rational human beings and not stereotyped nitwits, but more than 1.1 billion people all over the world are now prey to a tobacco addiction, especially when 78% of the smokers out there are men.

There is a rise of 3.4% consumption of tobacco in many countries, especially those which are developing, due to this excessive and extensive marketing campaign done by brands, which originated in countries where the smoking rate has fallen from 40% to 20% – UK and the United States!

Everybody knows about the harmful effects of a long-term tobacco usage and abuse. Nevertheless, man being man, he is going to persist on poisoning himself just for kicks.

So is not it time you kicked the butt right now, no pun intended. The tips given in this book are going to come in useful, under such circumstances.

Live Long, Live Healthy And Prosper!

Author Bio

Dueep Jyot Singh is a Management and IT Professional who managed to gather Postgraduate qualifications in Management and English and Degrees in Science, French and Education while pursuing different enjoyable career options like being an hospital administrator, IT,SEO and HRD Database Manager/ trainer, movie , radio and TV scriptwriter, theatre artiste and public speaker, lecturer in French, Marketing and Advertising, ex-Editor of Hearts On Fire (now known as Solstice) Books Missouri USA, advice columnist and cartoonist, publisher and Aviation School trainer, ex-moderator on Medico.in, banker, student councilor ,travelogue writer … among other things!

One fine morning, she decided that she had enough of killing herself by Degrees and went back to her first love -- writing. It's more enjoyable! She already has 48 published academic and 14 fiction- in- different- genre books under her belt.

When she is not designing websites or making Graphic design illustrations for clients , she is browsing through old bookshops hunting for treasures, of which she has an enviable collection – including R.L. Stevenson, O.Henry, Dornford Yates, Maurice Walsh, De Maupassant, Victor Hugo, Sapper, C.N. Williamson, "Bartimeus" and the crown of her collection- Dickens "The Old Curiosity Shop," and "Martin Chuzzlewit" and so on… Just call her "Renaissance Woman") - collecting herbal remedies, acting like Universal Helping Hand/Agony Aunt, or escaping to her dear mountains for a bit of exploring, collecting herbs and plants, and trekking.

Check out some of the other JD-Biz Publishing books

Gardening Series on Amazon

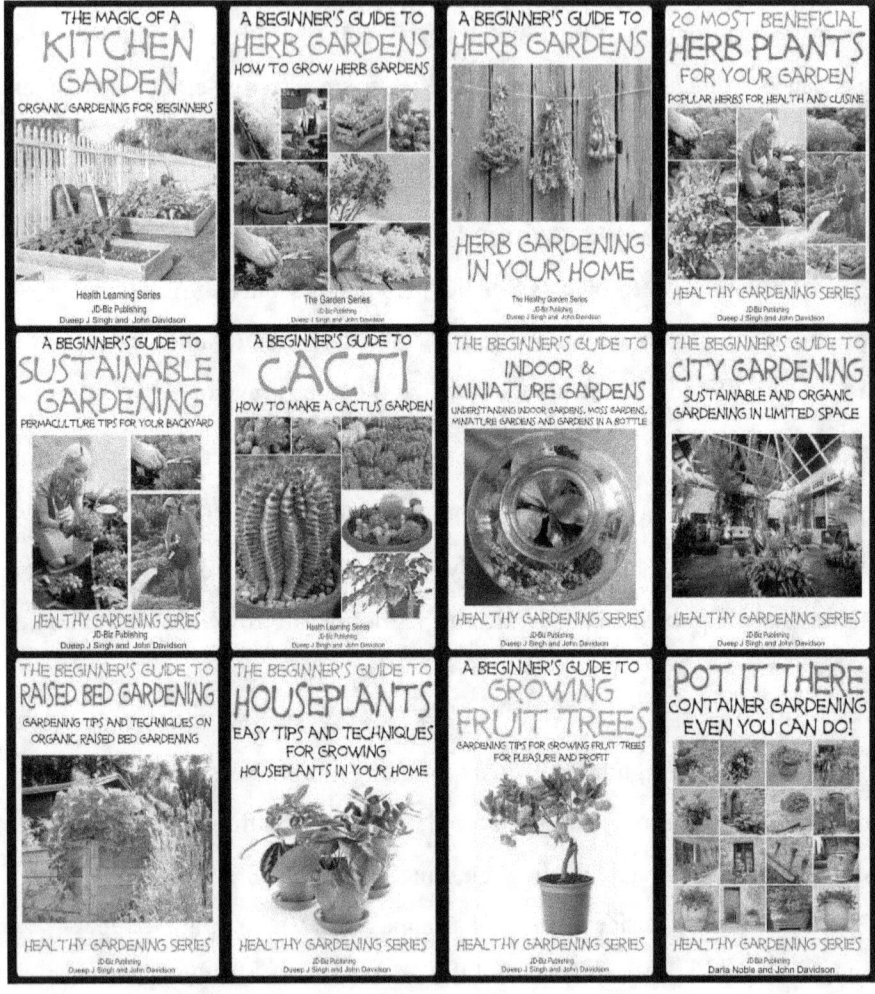

Health Learning Series

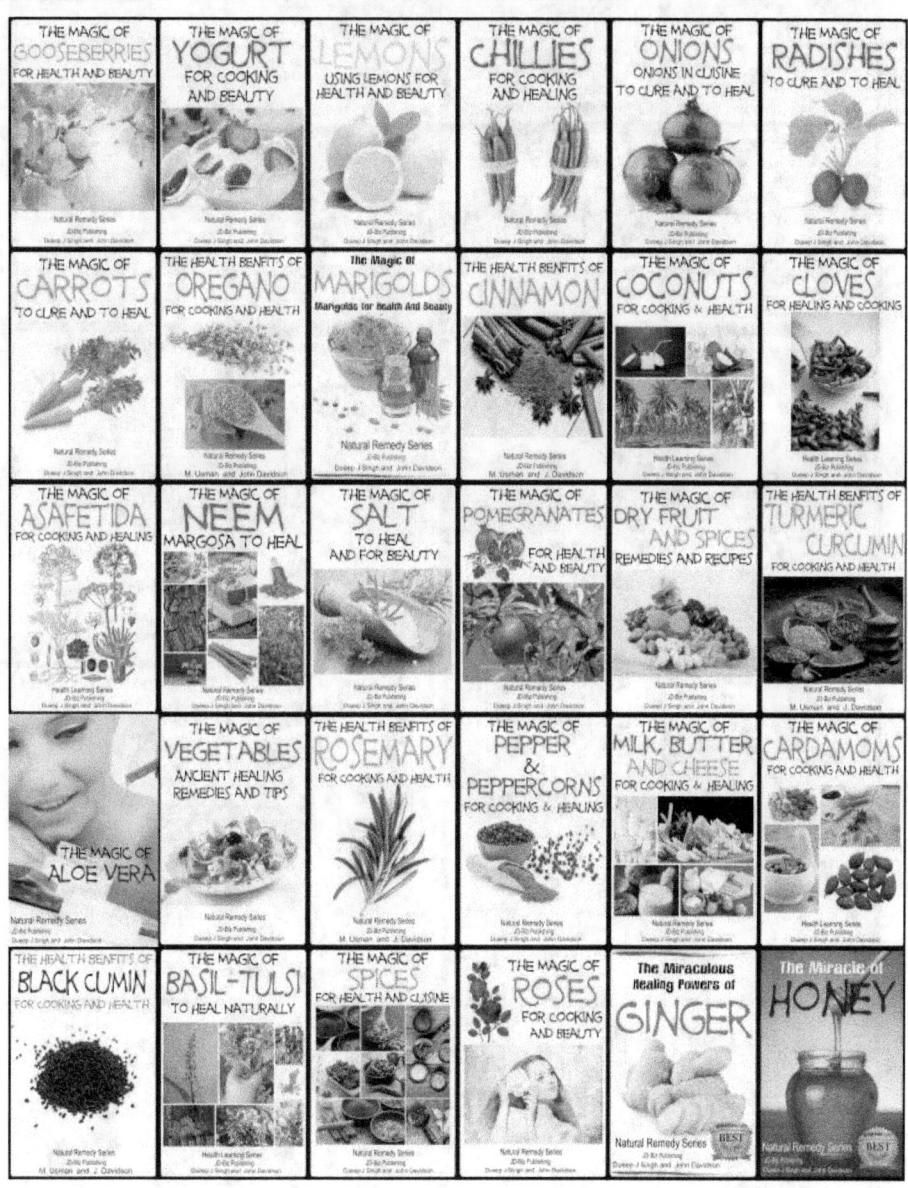

Country Life Books

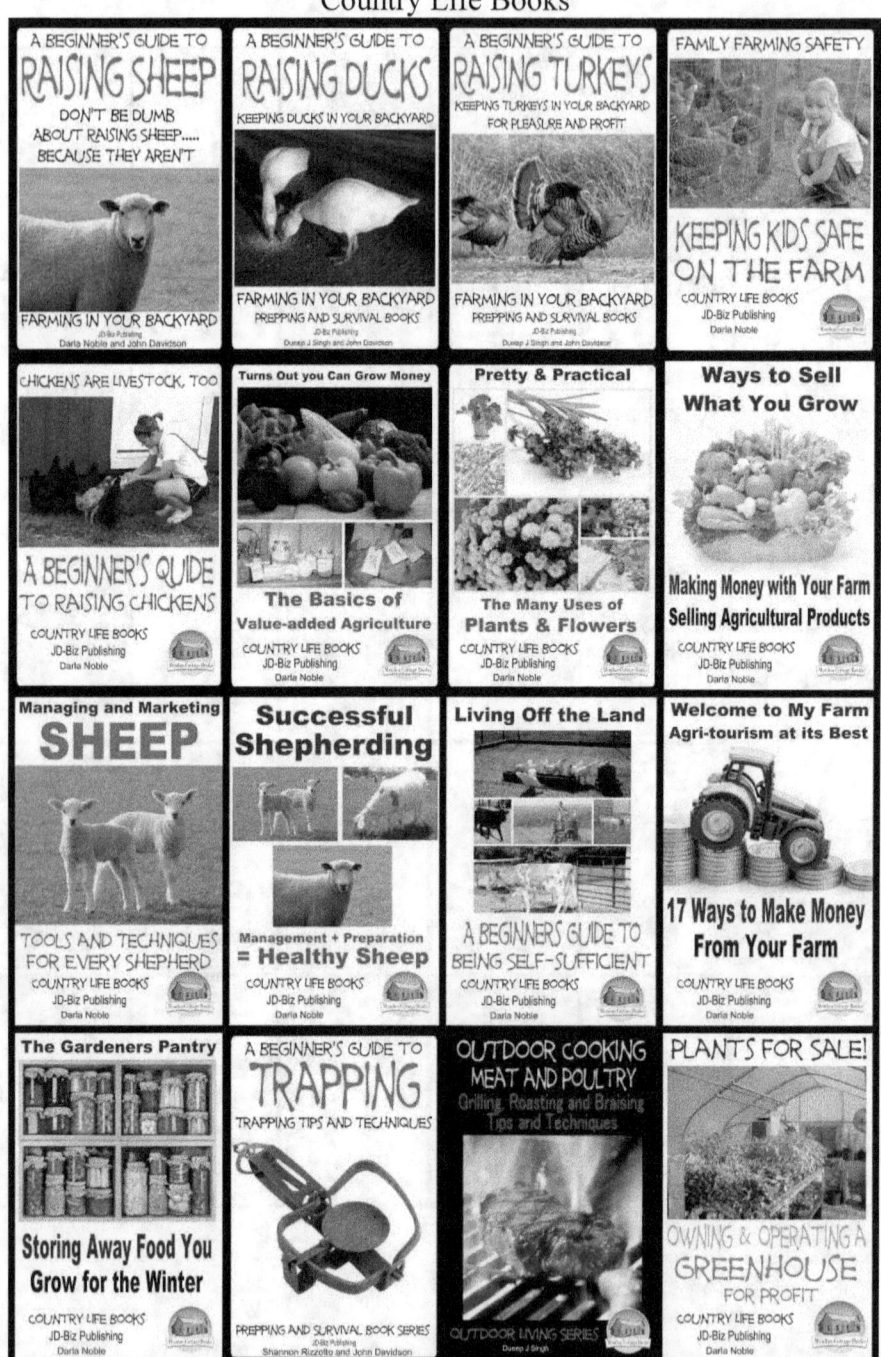

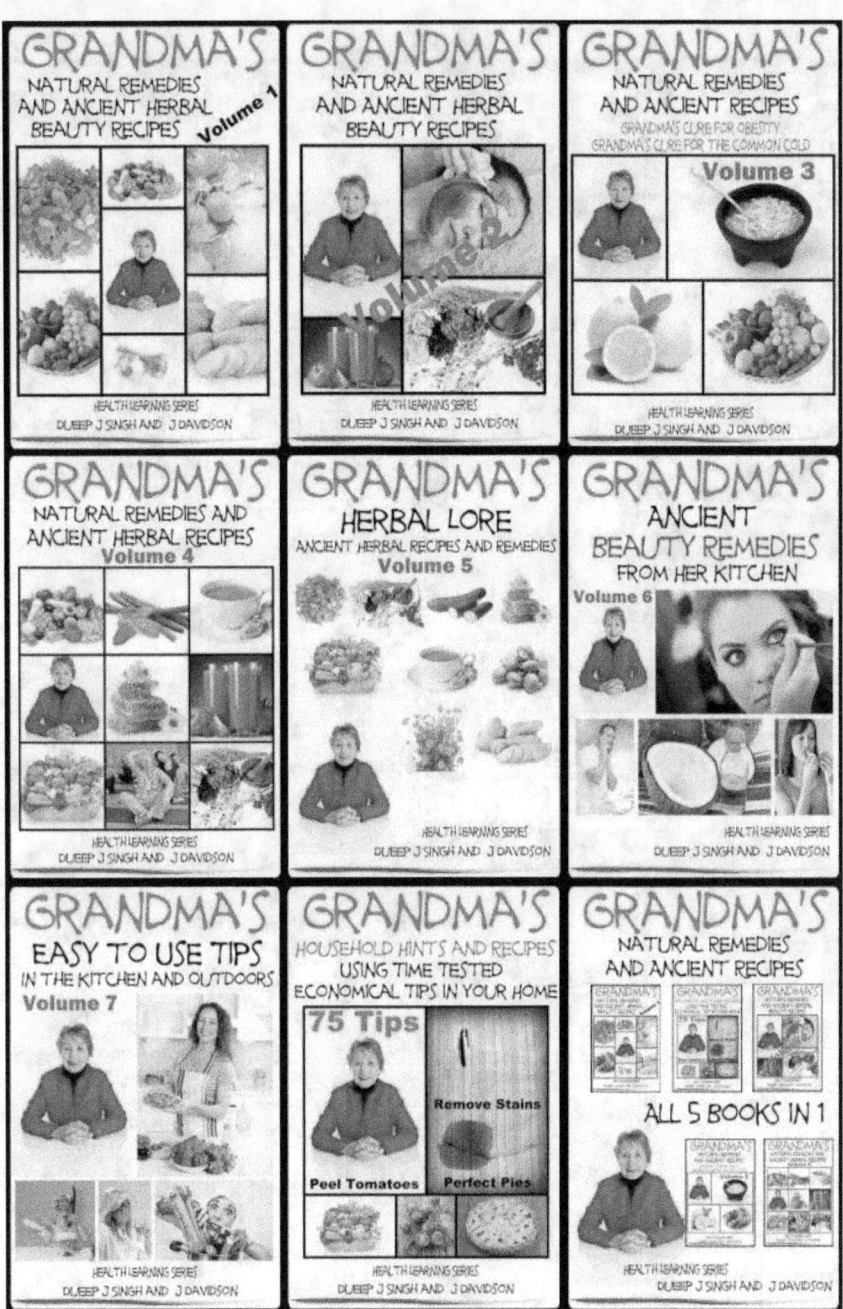

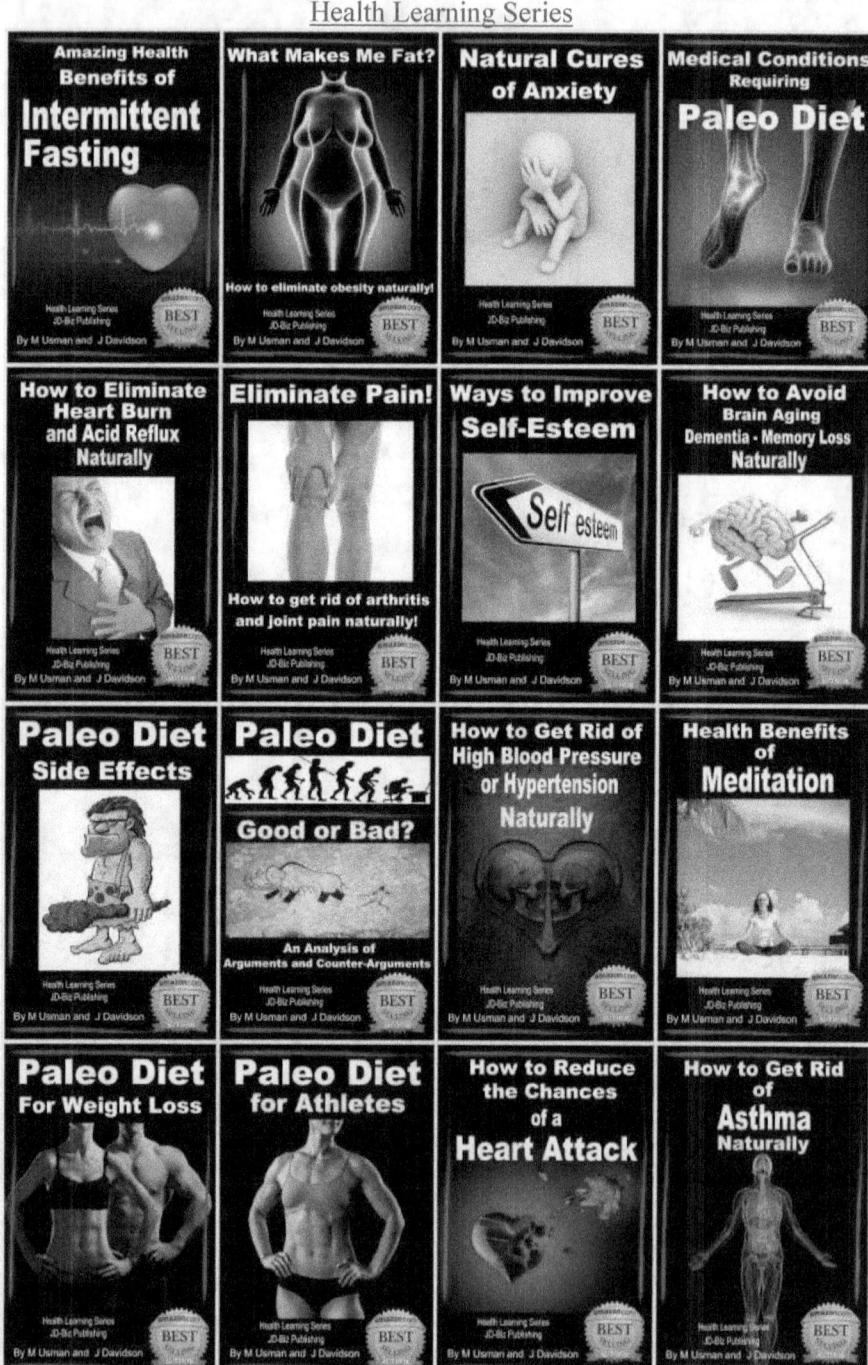

Amazing Animal Book Series

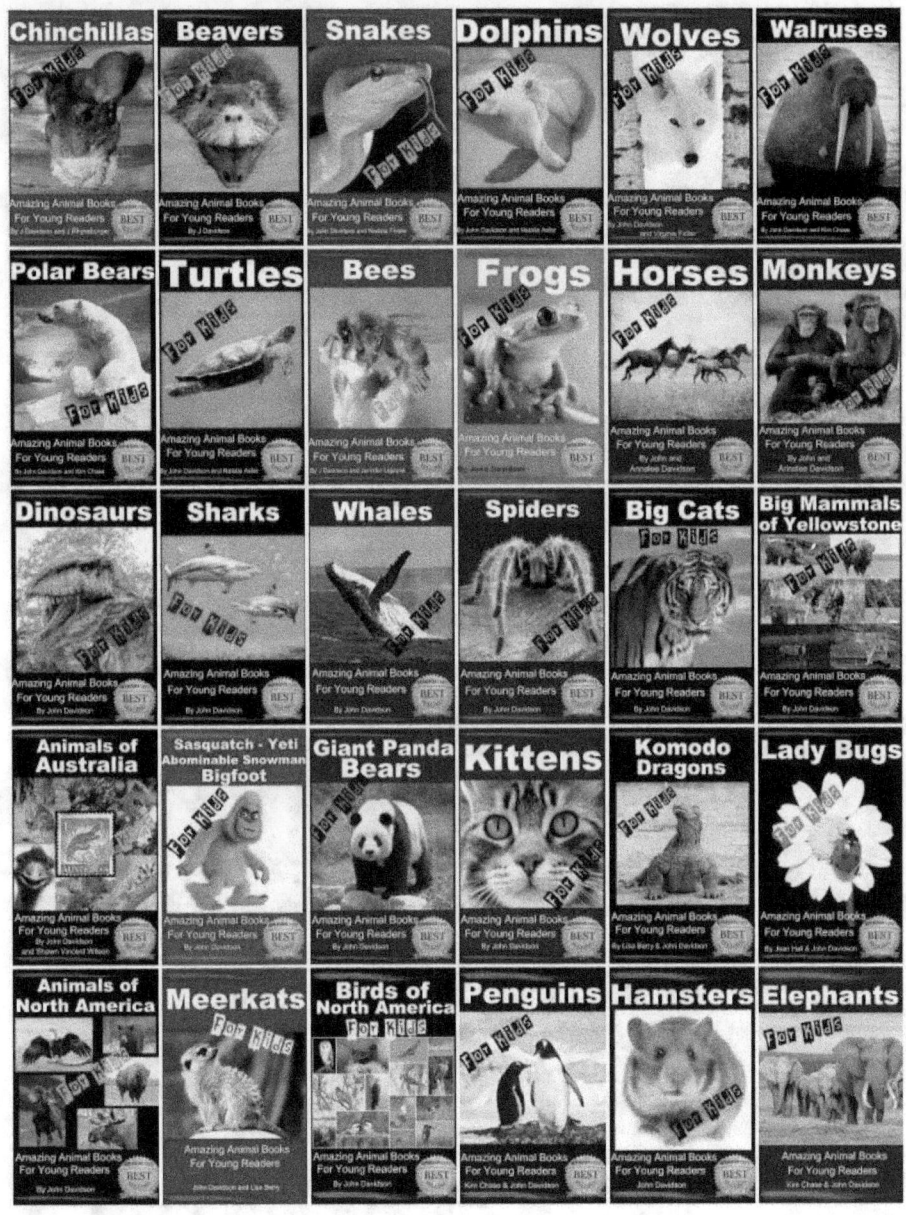

Learn To Draw Series

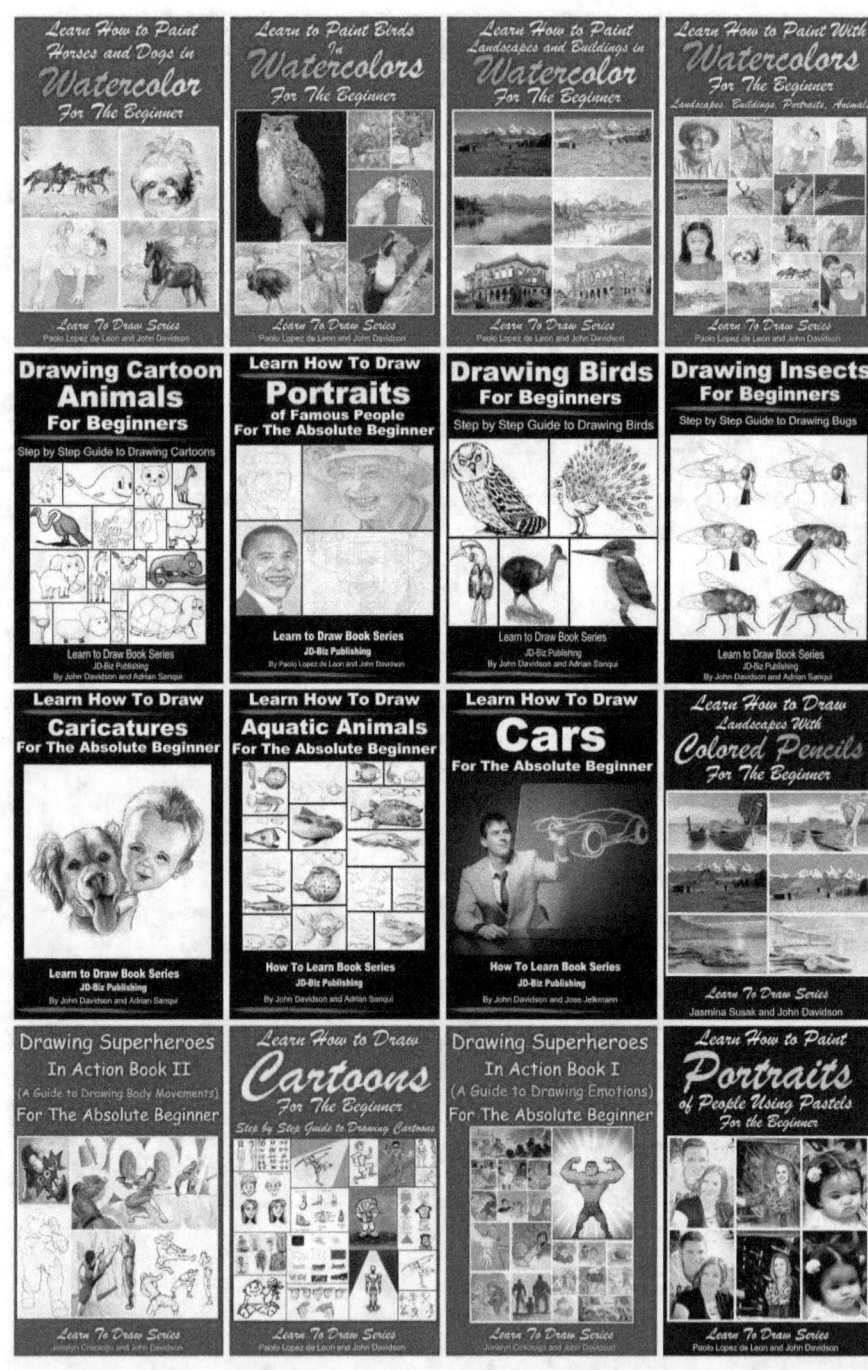

How to Build and Plan Books

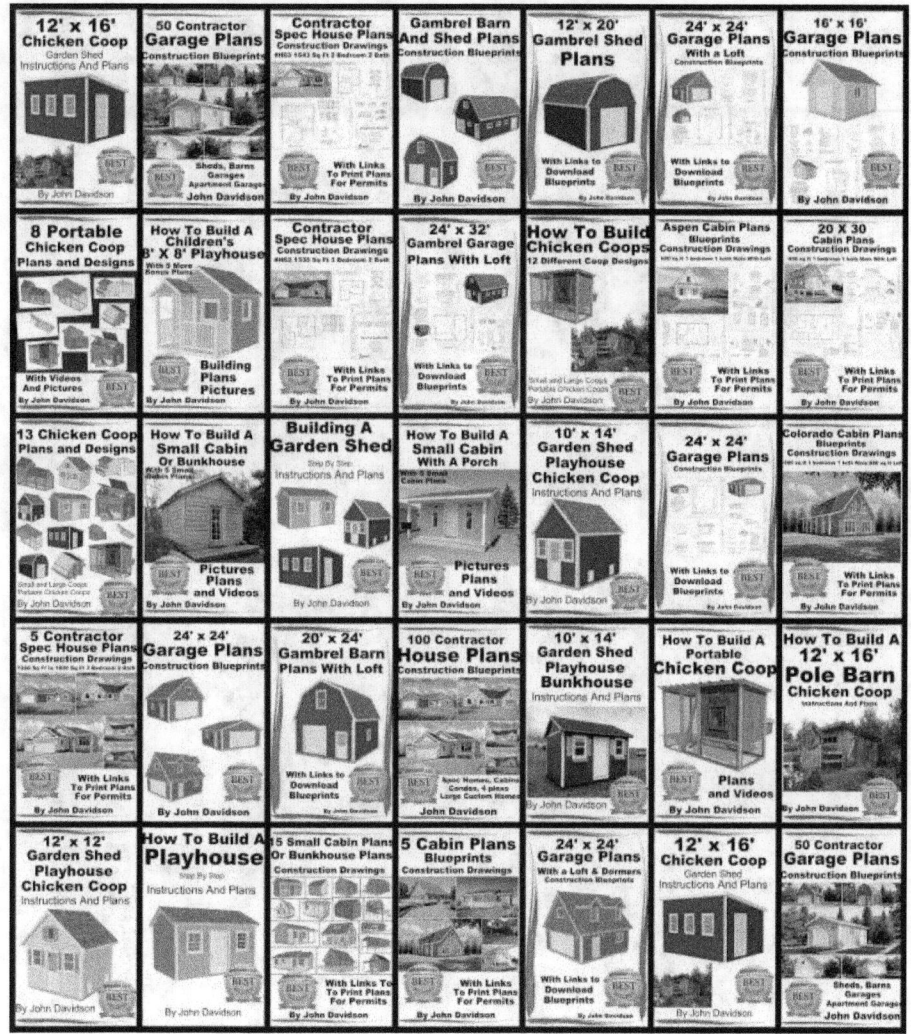

Entrepreneur Book Series

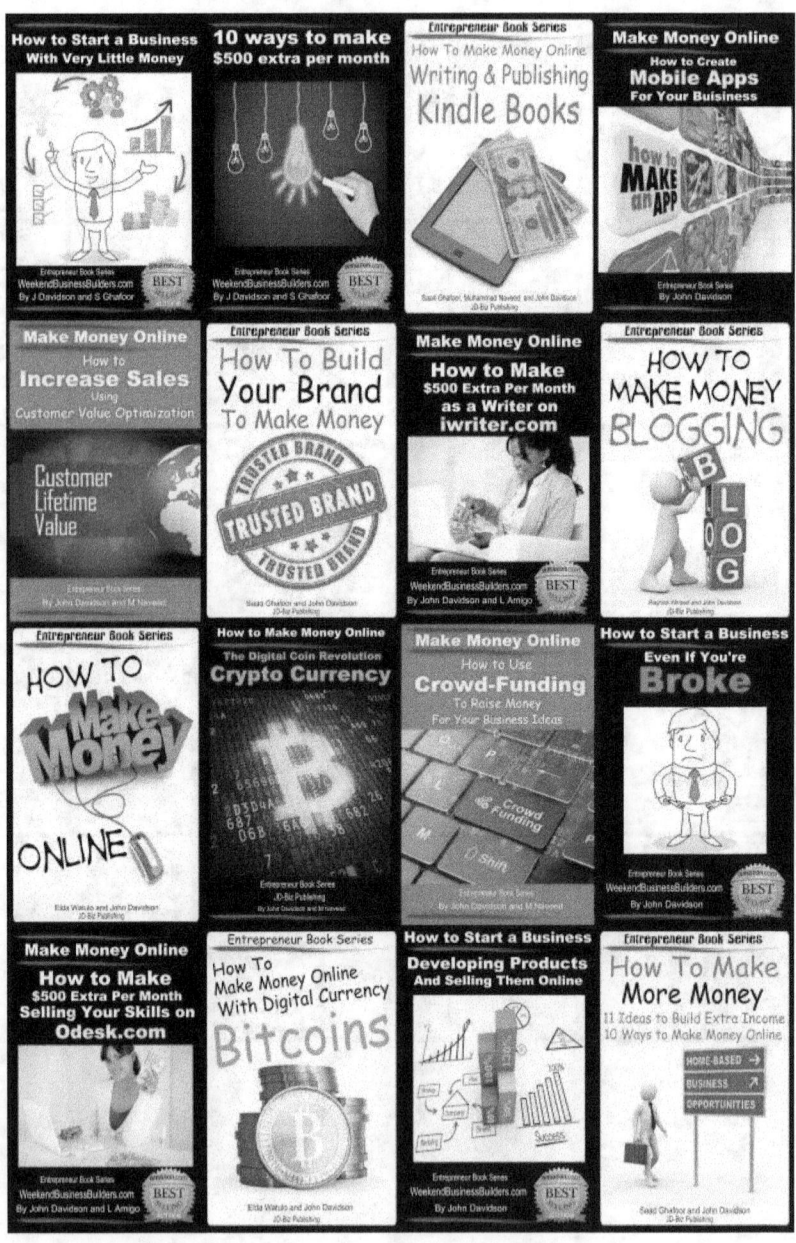

Our books are available at

1. Amazon.com

2. Barnes and Noble

3. Itunes

4. Kobo

5. Smashwords

6. Google Play Books

Publisher

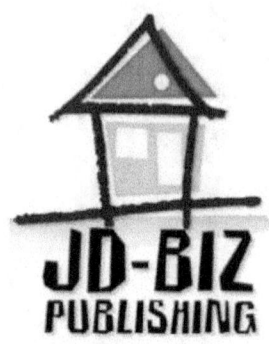

JD-Biz Corp

P O Box 374

Mendon, Utah 84325

http://www.jd-biz.com/

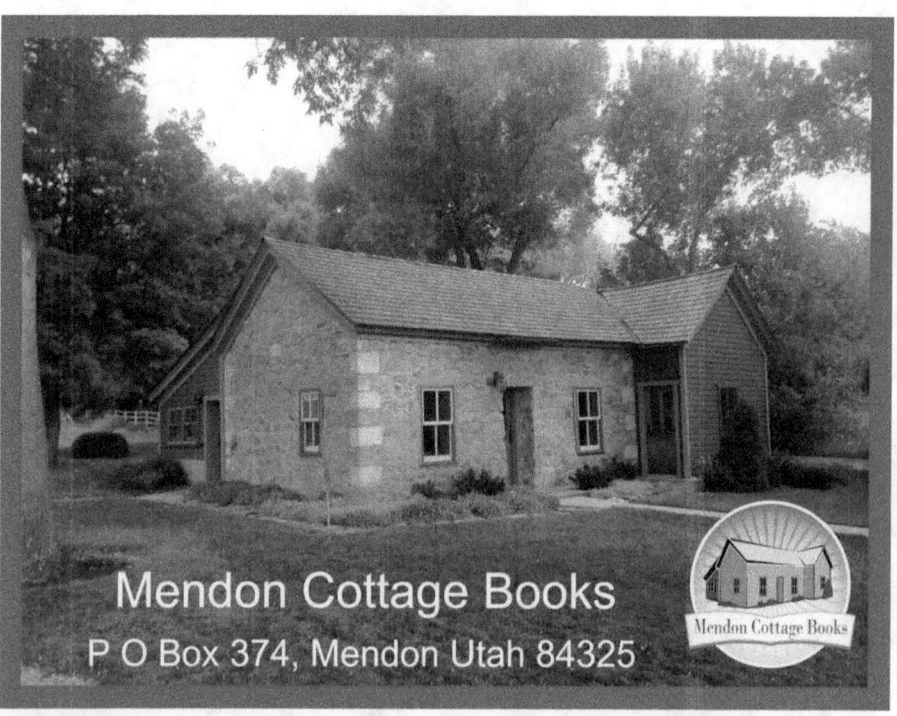

Mendon Cottage Books

P O Box 374, Mendon Utah 84325

www.ingramcontent.com/pod-product-compliance
Lightning Source LLC
Chambersburg PA
CBHW071235280526
45787CB00002B/940

* 9 7 8 1 5 1 7 1 9 9 5 0 0 *